THE TRUTH ABOUT BREASTFEEDING

—◆—

The Non-Judgmental Handbook
and Guide for Nursing Mothers

Alicia Chadwick

TABLE OF CONTENTS

——◆——

INTRODUCTION

—◆—

Motherhood is a unique journey that can be quite personal. Many women embark on this journey with a vague map that might illustrate important landmarks but lacks turn-by-turn directions to navigate those landmarks. Could you imagine having a GPS to navigate motherhood like you do to navigate traffic? It could give you updates on your route if an obstacle is up ahead and offer alternate routes, or it could let you know if some unforeseen incident is going to delay or speed up your journey.

Despite the strides made in public knowledge, no one has all the answers. I quickly discovered this after having and breastfeeding four children. I completely understand the rewards and trials that can come along with breastfeeding a baby, whether you're a new mother or a seasoned one. I have four vastly different breastfeeding experiences and wanted to share them to help other mothers.

Through my experiences, I am passionate about breastfeeding. If you're able to establish and sustain a successful breastfeeding relationship, you'll soon see the physical and emotional benefits firsthand. Not only is breast milk a complete source of nutrition for your baby, but breastfeeding can also have a positive impact on both the baby's and mother's physical and mental health.

I am in no way claiming to be an expert on breastfeeding (if you can ever be an expert in these sorts of things), but my advice comes from experience as opposed to certifications.

In the pages that follow, I'm going to share tips and tricks I've learned along the way and hopefully give you a nonjudgmental, safe place where you can mull over the ideas and suggestions I share that can really only come from experiencing them.

Whether you're picking this book up because your heart is set on breastfeeding or you're just looking for alternate options for feeding your baby, know that whatever you decide is the best choice for you and your baby. My goal is to support all mothers in any way they opt to feed their babies. I'm going to be providing tips and advice on breastfeeding, and you may decide that isn't what's best for you and your baby based on your season in life, which is completely understandable. I want you to feel empowered to make those decisions for your family. And those decisions can only be made when you have all the facts you can possibly gather.

So, while Motherhood GPS may not be a thing, consider this a travel brochure, giving you the highlights, things to look forward to, and the best ways to navigate unforeseen events that may crop up in your breastfeeding journey.

CHAPTER 1:

Motherhood's Most Natural Calling

—◆—

Breast milk is a biological response when your body becomes pregnant. It's natural and normal for your body to produce breast milk to nourish your baby. In fact, breast milk is complete in all the nutrients your baby needs for the first year of their life. Even with this proven knowledge, new mothers are often given conflicting information, making their decisions difficult to weigh.

The Weight of Expectation

If you ever want to see how quickly a woman can receive unsolicited advice, just watch her announce that she's expecting. For some reason, people (men and women alike) feel it necessary and appropriate to impart "wisdom" to expecting mothers. While some of this advice may be well-meaning and well intended, it is unasked for nonetheless. It can leave expecting mothers confused and scared.

Among some of the most damaging expectations are what is portrayed in the media. New mothers are often photographed in full makeup, looking well rested with a sleeping baby on their arm. If we could only all be so lucky. And advice from others can often damage our perception as well. I remember being told to "sleep when baby sleeps," which conveys the idea that babies sleep a lot, and we should take advantage of it. While it's true to some extent within those first few weeks back home, it's not always that simple. If the mother has a partner in the home, oftentimes that partner has to continue to work once the baby arrives, which leaves Mom feeling like she has to resume her maternal duties while her partner is at work. It can feel overwhelming as you struggle between sleeping while the baby sleeps or throwing a load of laundry in the washer to try and hack away at the growing mountain of dirty clothes. I remember trying to reason with myself in those first months: "I'll just throw this in the washer, then get something to eat, and then I'll lie down." But before I could close my eyes, the baby was stirring again. As with most advice, it's nice in theory. But unfortunately, that just isn't always our reality. Not to mention the fact that so much of those first few months is responding to your baby's ever-changing cues and demands. As soon as you feel like you've fallen into a rhythm and routine, something will come along to disrupt it, may it be teething, illness, or new milestones.

Some mothers may also find themselves torn with the type of parent they want to be. Before I had children, I wanted to develop an attachment style of parenting that was responsive to my child's needs. I wanted to create a safe and loving environment in which I built my baby's trust and gave them the room to explore the world around them. But often, I was met with resistance from those who felt as though I was allowing my child to rule my life. They were the same people who advocated for stringent routines and expectations. But what happens when those stringent routines and expectations don't work for you? Alexander Pope once wrote: "Blessed is he who expects nothing, for he shall never be disappointed" (Pope, 1727). When we build up our expectations for the way something should be, we are profoundly disappointed when it doesn't work out the way we had hoped. I'm not saying you should go into parenthood with no expectations or expecting the worst. Rather, approach it with a more laid-back attitude if possible. When you look at your child, give yourself grace and allow yourself to be flexible despite what other people might think.

Influence of Inner Circles

Typically, our greatest source of support (or judgment) can come from those closest to us. Ideally, our close friends and family would seek to support us as we embark on this new endeavor. As with unsolicited advice from strangers, the same can come from those within our inner circles. My family assumed I would breastfeed, and while that was what I wanted to do, the expectation presented its own pressure. What if I wasn't able to successfully breastfeed my baby for some reason? I felt guilty for even considering the possibility of using formula. I think that trying to adhere to the standards of what you should or shouldn't be doing as set forth by those closest to you can actually be more damaging to your immediate family unit. Let's say Aunt Fran is telling you to put baby on a schedule. You attempt it, but it just ends the same way every day. Then, frustration, when things don't go to plan, dissolves into unresolved anger, which can morph into you and your partner taking your anger out on each other because you're frustrated and potentially not getting sleep.

I am a huge proponent of doing what's easiest for you and your family, especially in the early days. Take the path of least resistance as you navigate this new world with your tiny new baby. You don't owe anyone an explanation for the lifestyle you choose. If they offer advice, you can simply smile and nod and possibly file their advice away to dissect later. Maybe there are some useful caveats. But don't be afraid to stand your ground and do what works for you and your baby. Additionally, if someone asks about your breastfeeding experience or sleeping arrangements, you can simply offer that you're doing what works for you and your baby. Or you can say that everything is so new, but you and baby are getting to know each other and learning what works for each of you. Typically, if you share your struggles, people often see that as an opportunity to offer unsolicited advice. Consider only sharing those struggles with those whose advice you value or who you know is more aligned with the type of parenting you're striving to achieve.

Managing Guilt and Judgment

One thing that doesn't get said when new mothers are expecting is, "Welcome to motherhood, where guilt and judgment will likely plague you for the rest of your life." Doesn't exactly sell the gift of motherhood, does it? While it is a harsh reality, it's also only one side of the coin. Motherhood is an incredibly beautiful station that is one of the most amazing things to me about being a human. You create this life inside of you, foster its health and growth for nine months, and usher it into this world, promising to keep it safe and cared for. You then go on to develop one of the deepest relationships you'll likely ever have with another person. A breastfeeding mother is usually well in tune with their baby; you learn to interpret their cues, cries, and moods and respond accordingly.

While motherhood is incredibly beautiful and awe-inspiring, it also comes with its own set of challenges. As mentioned above, it seems that everyone has an opinion on how or when women breastfeed. From breastfeeding in public to how long you choose to breastfeed, these topics garner varying supporters on both sides. Public breastfeeding is one thing that seems to be a hot topic. I blame the sexualization of a woman's body on the perception of breastfeeding in public. Breasts have come to symbolize sexuality, so when a woman attempts to breastfeed in public, some people are unable to separate their preconceived notion from the fact that the mother is not committing a sexual act, but rather she's feeding her baby. So, unfortunately, many women will be shamed or judged for breastfeeding in public.

This judgment and shame can weigh heavily on mothers. Instead of focusing on doing what is right for herself and her baby, a mother's focus may shift to avoid scrutiny as an act of self-preservation. Providing the basic needs for a baby is exhausting on its own; throw in managing judgment and shame, and you have one emotionally and physically exhausted momma.

This judgment and shame can be further aggravated if hurdles with breastfeeding arise and Mom finds herself in a position where she's struggling to provide the basic nutrients for her baby. Some may question why something so natural is so difficult for her. This may lead to the mom questioning her ability and skill as a mother.

But something you need to know is that motherhood and breastfeeding are *hard*. It is fraught with challenges. Even if you're a mother of multiple children, no two children are the same. My oldest child was a textbook baby when it came to sleeping patterns and breastfeeding. But my second child? Oh boy, he came with a bunch of hurdles we had to learn how to overcome! So, what worked with my oldest didn't always work as well with my younger child.

You just have to do your best to shove the expectations and judgment of society and your inner circle out of your mind. We have a hard enough job as it is, and chances are, you're harder on yourself than anyone else will ever be. Remind yourself that your body was built for this, and you were gifted your child for a reason. At your base intuition, you know what is best for you and your baby. If that means skipping Great-Aunt Gertrude's birthday in favor of getting more rest, that's what you need to do. Or maybe that means allowing your baby to breastfeed themselves to sleep despite what your mother thinks that will do to your baby in the long term. No one else has to live with you and your baby. Only you can make the best decisions for you as you learn what does and doesn't work for you and your baby. Sure, you can take what people tell you with a grain of salt, but don't take it to heart. Sift through their advice and "words of wisdom" and pluck out the gems you think might be worth stowing away for later. But remember, you brought this baby into the world and nurtured them for nine months on *your body alone*, so if anyone is an expert on your baby, it's you!

CHAPTER 2:

Mommy's Milk

—◆—

The human body is truly magnificent, especially when it comes to growing and nourishing another human! From conception to birth to postnatal life, a mother's body is perfectly designed to provide everything her baby needs.

The Science Behind Milk Production

Once you become pregnant, hormones in your body (elevated levels of progesterone and estrogen) signal the need for lactation. The process of lactation is known as lactogenesis and begins around the sixteenth week of pregnancy. However, your body doesn't immediately begin making breast milk. Within the breast are alveoli and milk ducts, which are essential to the process of breastfeeding. It can be helpful to imagine the components of breastfeeding as a tree. The nipple is the tree trunk, the milk ducts can be seen as the branches, and the alveoli would be considered the leaves.

The first thing to happen with the onset of lactogenesis is that your milk ducts will grow in number and size. Many women will note that their breasts become fuller during pregnancy, and that can be attributed to the growth of their milk ducts. The body will begin to produce colostrum. This is the early days of breastmilk, which your body will produce until your baby is born.

Once your baby is born (and the placenta is delivered), those hormones that signal your body to begin making breast milk (progesterone and estrogen) will drop, and another hormone, prolactin, will increase. This signals your body to intensify milk production. It can take up to three days for your milk to come in following the birth of your baby. Until your milk comes in, the colostrum is enough to sustain your newborn baby.

The Key to Efficient Feeding

Breastfeeding Basics

Breastfeeding is based solely on supply and demand. As long as milk is being removed from the breast, your body will make more. The breast is a responsive body part in the act of breastfeeding. It's important to latch your baby onto your breast as soon as possible following birth. It's also important to note your baby's mouth should be coming in contact with and stimulating the areola in addition to the nipple. The areola is comprised of sensitive nerve endings. When these nerve endings are stimulated by your baby's mouth, it signals to your body to release milk from the alveoli to the ducts. Your nipple contains about twenty pores in which the milk is released for your baby.

As mentioned above, the areola and nipple are important components of the breastfeeding system. Not only does baby's suckling provide your body with information that results in milk being released, but your baby's saliva actually interacts with your breast and sends signals to your body, indicating baby's immunological needs. Understandably, some mothers will ask if they should breastfeed while they're sick. If you take any medications, it's best to consult with your doctor to ensure there isn't any danger to your baby. But if there isn't any danger, it's actually highly recommended to breastfeed your baby while you're sick if you're able. Even if you don't feel comfortable having them in close proximity, providing them with your expressed breast milk can be beneficial as well. When you become sick, your body produces antibodies that are passed through your breast milk, providing baby with their first line of defense. Additionally, your baby can't get sick simply by breastfeeding. Germs can be spread in the other ways they normally are (airborne or through exchanging fluid, like if you kiss your baby), but your baby isn't at risk of contracting an illness you have just because they consume your breastmilk.

Letdown Reflex

When your baby is able to latch properly onto your breast, their suckling motion stimulates the areolas as well as the nipple. It signals the body to release prolactin and oxytocin. The prolactin sends a signal to the alveoli to make more milk, while the oxytocin produces muscle contractions that aid in pushing milk out of the alveoli through the milk ducts. When this happens, this is known as your "letdown." Oftentimes, your letdown can be accompanied by a tingling sensation in the breasts. This isn't always the case, but it can be just one physical indication that your milk is letting down. The letdown reflex can take a minute or two to kick in once baby latches and begins stimulating the nipple and areola. You may notice your baby's sucking pattern change once your letdown happens. Since the milk is flowing more freely, they may not need to suckle in the same manner to withdraw milk.

It's not uncommon to experience two or three letdowns in one breastfeeding session.

Some moms experience overactive letdown. This happens when your milk aggressively exits the pores in your nipple without much effort required from your baby (if at all). You may experience leaking from the breast your baby is not feeding from if you have an overactive letdown. Additionally, depending on how aggressively your milk comes out, your baby may appear to be struggling while at the breast during your initial letdown. If that's the case, consider inserting your pinkie finger into your baby's mouth to dislodge them from your breast and remove them from your breast to allow the initial letdown to pass. Once you feel as though it's not as strong, you can replace your baby on the breast, and they can resume feeding.

You may encounter an instance in which you want to trigger a letdown. Some women will have a recording of their baby cooing or crying if they need to express while apart from their baby. Sometimes, even just thinking of your baby can encourage the letdown reflex. If you're with your baby and struggling to have a letdown, consider ensuring that you're completely relaxed. Sometimes, when you're tensed and stressed, your body will respond by locking down what might come naturally. As you're breastfeeding, pay attention to your shoulders. If they're bunched up by your ears, relax your shoulders and the rest of your body. As you make sure your body is relaxed, also concentrate on your breathing. If you're stressed about stuff around the home, consider asking your partner, friend, or family member to lend a hand so you can focus on feeding your baby.

As long as milk is being removed from the breast, your body will replenish it. If, for some reason, you have to be separated from your baby for any length of time that might span a feeding, consider expressing milk as though they were feeding so your body is prompted to continue with milk production.

Night Feeding

Think for a moment about your sleep habits. Do you often sleep through the night without waking? I'm willing to bet you don't. When I first had my oldest child, I was presented with this question, and it changed how I viewed the desire to have my baby sleep through the night. If we, as adults, are prone to waking up throughout the night due to thirst, a bad dream, or having to use the bathroom, why would our babies be any different?

Additionally, when your baby was growing in your belly, they were used to having regular, unfettered access to nutrition through the umbilical cord. When you think about the cozy environment your uterus provides, their transition into the world can be viewed as a jarring one. They went from a controlled, comfortable, muted environment to one with overwhelming sights, sounds, and feelings. In addition to acclimating to all that, they need to get used to not being continuously fed anymore.

New mothers are often asked if baby is sleeping through the night as an indicator of whether their baby is "good." But this oft-asked question is misinformed at best and judgmental at worst. This "innocent" question perpetuates the myth that babies will face long-term sleep issues if they're not sleeping through the night by a certain point. That's just not the case. Babies wake through the night for a myriad of reasons, just like adults do. Especially within the first few months of baby's life, it's not uncommon for baby to frequently nurse from nine p.m. to three a.m. on and off. They can receive approximately twenty percent of their caloric needs in that time frame! So, trying to put baby on a schedule and regulate them within the first six months can be detrimental to their development.

If you attempt to put baby on a nighttime feeding schedule they're not ready for, this may lead to weight loss for them and a reduction in milk supply for you. As mentioned previously, breast milk is replenished when the current supply is expressed. So, if you cut down on night feedings in favor of a routine, your body may think the baby is weaning off breast milk, and will reduce the amount of milk your body is making.

Night feedings ensure adequate supply, foster the mother and baby relationship, and promote healthy physical and mental development for your baby.

You may notice your baby fall into a more predictable rhythm after a few months, but then, all of a sudden, your baby's night feedings seem to increase again. A baby may increase feedings (particularly nighttime feedings) for any number of reasons, which can include a growth spurt, teething, or a developmental milestone.

Another common myth is that breastfed babies will wake more often than babies who receive formula. Regardless of the means of nutrition, babies will wake frequently throughout the night. In fact, breastfed mothers have been found to get better sleep than mothers who formula-feed. This can be attributed to the prolactin your body releases when you're breastfeeding. Additionally, when a baby is fed formula, the formula has to be prepared. With breastfeeding mothers, the baby can be put on the breast without having to fully wake up, which results in having an easier time falling back asleep once baby is done nursing.

Waking up throughout the night can be tiresome and difficult to get used to, but if you're breastfeeding, consider making it easier on yourself. If you have baby in a different room, place a bassinet in your room so you can be more easily roused when your baby begins to stir for their night feeding. This also provides the benefit that baby isn't getting too worked up to get your attention. If the baby is in a different room, they may completely wake up indicating they're hungry, so now they need to be soothed before they're fed. Sleeping in the same room not only increases the ease of breastfeeding, but your baby's body also tunes in to your circadian rhythm. So when your baby starts to wake for a night feeding, chances are you won't be in as deep of a sleep, and it'll be easier for you to wake up and tend to them.

You can also ask your partner to lend a hand at night to take some of the stress off you. If you're waking the baby to feed them, consider asking your partner to handle diaper duty if baby needs their diaper changed.

The first few months of baby's life will be a brand-new world for you and them. Give yourself grace and follow your baby's cues. It can be difficult, but whatever works for you and your baby is best. You may find you try multiple different options to discover this, and that's normal.

Breastfeeding After Surgery

Women may find themselves needing breast surgery, and this may raise concerns about whether they will be able to breastfeed in the future. Your best bet is to discuss your future wishes and concerns with your doctor. Make them aware of your desire to breastfeed, and ask them if the surgery will impact that in the future. Unfortunately, there are no guarantees, but generally, doctors can provide an educated guess based on previous cases and experiences.

If you're receiving a breast augmentation (or have received one previously), breastfeeding is absolutely within the realm of possibility for you—whether the augmentation was made over or under the muscle. It's important to talk to your doctor about any concerns you have and ask questions. The main concern with breast augmentation and breastfeeding is the possibility of the implant aggravating or causing engorgement and impacting their ability to fully empty the milk ducts. To prevent discomfort and encourage continued milk production, it's recommended to empty the breasts as often as possible if you notice this in your breastfeeding relationship. If you're feeling engorged before baby is due for their next feeding, consider expressing (either by hand or with a mechanical pump) enough milk to relieve the discomfort. This milk can be saved and stored for baby at a later time in the event that you need to be away from baby for any reason during one of their feedings.

On the other hand, if you had breast reduction surgery, breastfeeding may be less likely for you. Part of the breast's structure includes the milk ducts, and as part of the removal of some of the breast tissue, it's very likely milk ducts are removed with a breast reduction. It's not to say breastfeeding is impossible; it just reduces the likelihood. If you are able to breastfeed following a breast reduction, you may find yourself needing to feed baby more frequently than your counterparts who have not undergone a breast reduction. As with any procedure, it's important to discuss your wishes with your doctor and explore possibilities and potential outcomes.

I have had friends who have had breast augmentation as well as reduction and have been able to successfully breastfeed their babies. While some caution may need to be exercised, don't let these things make you think you can't breastfeed at all.

New mothers are often inundated with outdated advice, inappropriate questions, and judgment from friends, family, and even strangers. If you find yourself experiencing any of this, remind yourself that you know your baby better than anyone. Your body grew and nourished that baby for nine months, and only you have an intimate knowledge of their body, cues, and needs. At the end of the day, trust your instincts. You have to live with your baby and the choices you make for them. You don't owe anyone an explanation or justification for the decisions you make when they're made with your baby's well-being in mind. You're doing a fantastic job; keep it up, Momma!

CHAPTER 3:

Your First Line of Defense

—◆—

Have you ever heard the old adage "Preparation is the key to success"? This can be applied to breastfeeding as much as it can be applied to any other aspect of your life. No, you can't adequately prepare for every possible situation that may arise as you establish the breastfeeding relationship with your baby, but having some of the essentials on hand will potentially increase your ease of breastfeeding and ensure your success. During your pregnancy, it may be helpful to make purchases that can sustain successful breastfeeding.

Essential Supplies for Breastfeeding

Once I had my baby, I found that leaking breast milk was a real concern, especially in the early days. Some women experience slight leaking of their breasts as they near their due date, so it may be a good idea to look at buying breast pads before baby arrives. Before I had my first baby, I was given disposable breast pads as a gift, and I was extremely thankful for it! If you don't notice your breasts leaking colostrum before delivery, you can still purchase different breast pads to find the ones that are the most comfortable for you.

Breast pads are worn inside the bra in front of the nipple. They absorb any milk that escapes so you aren't leaking into your bra or through your shirt, which can save you from embarrassment or an impromptu outfit change. As mentioned, leaking can happen in the early days as you're establishing your milk supply, and it's also common to leak during a letdown; this can happen if you experience a letdown unexpectedly or if you're breastfeeding. It's common for the breast baby is not feeding from to leak during a letdown.

Thankfully, you have options to look into when it comes to breast pads.

Disposable breast pads are typically made of a thin, absorbent material and often come with an adhesive that can be placed on the bra. This keeps the pad in place as you move around throughout the day.

Reusable breast pads are a great option if you don't want to continuously purchase disposable pads. They don't often have any type of adhesive on the back side, but since they're made from fabric, they don't usually slip around like a disposable pad would be prone to do. The reusable pads are generally constructed with several layers to ensure the pad absorbs any leaks, but these layers are highly absorbent and not typically thick or bulky. Depending on how much you leak, the pad can generally be worn throughout the day and will need to be washed afterward. Reusable pads are a good option if you have sensitive skin and notice your breast or nipple having an adverse reaction to disposable pads.

Disposable pads can generally be easily found at most big-box stores that sell breastfeeding and baby essentials. Some may also sell reusable breast pads, but those are most commonly sold online from specialty or boutique stores.

In addition to breast pads, nursing bras might be a good item to look at before your baby is born. As mentioned previously, when you become pregnant, you may notice your breasts changing. They may become larger and more tender. Breastfeeding may be the furthest thing from your mind, but as you look to acquire more comfortable clothes, don't discount a good nursing bra. Yes, a nursing bra's main purpose is to increase the ease of breastfeeding. They're also generally more comfortable than your average bra. So, instead of going out and buying new regular bras, start looking for comfortable nursing bras. However, a good rule of thumb is to avoid buying a nursing bra too early into your pregnancy. I was given the advice to wait until my third trimester to purchase a nursing bra because your breasts can change so much during pregnancy with fluctuations in hormones. Once you're in your third trimester, your pregnancy hormones will continue to fluctuate, but not nearly as much. Additionally, when looking for a nursing bra, consider avoiding ones with underwire. It may be tempting to purchase an underwire nursing bra, but the underwire can dig into the breast tissue and inhibit your body's effectiveness at expelling milk. Not to mention, the underwire may be uncomfortable against your likely tender breasts. Thankfully, there are many options to consider when shopping for nursing bras. They can be found at many big box stores, but there are also stores that specialize in maternity wear that can guide you on the ones that can provide you with the best support and comfort.

Take the time before baby comes to shop for accessories that will increase your comfort. If possible, buy a couple of different items of the same thing (two different brands of nursing bras, for example) to see which will be more comfortable for you.

Maternity Wear and Dual-Purpose Clothing

Once you become pregnant, you'll soon discover that comfort is key. As mentioned above, your breasts will begin to change, and the rest of your body will follow soon after. The more obvious indication of pregnancy (a growing belly) will make your current wardrobe uncomfortable after a couple of months. Maternity clothes are known for growing with you throughout your pregnancy. And the best part? You can continue to wear those clothes once you deliver your baby. Despite what is often portrayed in the media, your body will not deflate as soon as the baby comes out. I remember being surprised with my first baby when I still looked pregnant when I left the hospital! But it makes sense if you think about the fact that your body just spent months rearranging itself to accommodate your growing baby. It's going to take time for everything to resettle where it once was. And you may find that some things don't resettle at all. But that's not abnormal. Once you have a baby, it's not uncommon for your body to look different.

Beyond the outward physical changes in your body, your body is also pumping extra blood through your veins, typically at a slightly elevated rate. Can you think about what happens when your blood is pumping faster through your body? Usually, your body temperature increases. Maternity wear is often made of stretchy material that breathes, so as you feel yourself fluctuating between hold and cold, maternity clothes will allow your skin to breathe, resulting in you likely feeling overheated due to your clothing. Once you deliver the baby, your body will be working to adjust to the drastic hormone changes. This may result in discomfort from varying temperatures as well. The breathable maternity clothes you wear during your pregnancy will aid your comfort as you heal postpartum as well.

As you look to add to your wardrobe, consider your comfort foremost. Leggings or jeans with a built-in stretchy panel are amazing throughout pregnancy and postpartum. The stretchy material isn't only comfortable because it grows with you, but it also typically has support that will give you relief with your growing belly. Aches and discomfort in your groin and stomach area are common throughout pregnancy, and just like a supportive bra is important for your breasts, a supportive pair of pants can help alleviate some of that discomfort.

Second-hand bargains can be found online and in second-hand stores or sales. Many women sell their hardly worn maternity clothes in great condition. But just know that you'll definitely get your money's worth for the clothes you purchase during pregnancy if you continue to wear them into postpartum!

In addition to looking to buy new clothes for your wardrobe, consider looking at what you already have in your closet. Some clothes can continue to be worn while you're pregnant and breastfeeding. If you have loose-fitting or oversized shirts, those are great to accommodate your growing belly. Also, if you're pregnant during the warmer seasons, flowy dresses that are looser fitting in the waist can be very comfortable despite not being traditional maternity wear. Exercise pants are another article of clothing that may be worn into your pregnancy as the material is often stretchy and comfortable. So before you panic about needing all new clothes, take a peek at what you have that you can make work while you're pregnant.

Handy Tools for Breastfeeding Preparation

Begin to explore some of the tools that may make your breastfeeding journey easier. Thankfully, there are many options available, but as you dive into what is out there, keep in mind that not all of it is necessary.

For me, an essential part of my breastfeeding arsenal is a breast pump. Even if you are planning to exclusively breastfeed, you may find it useful to have one on hand. You can use it to express milk when you're engorged for whatever reason, if you and your spouse want to enjoy a date night, or if you plan on returning to work at some point.

There are various models available for purchase, but you don't need the most elite and expensive one. Mechanical and manual breast pumps are available, and if you will only need one from time to time, a manual breast pump may be all you need. Having a breast pump available allows for flexibility and options to express milk while you're breastfeeding your baby.

In addition to a breast pump, you'll need milk storage bags and bottles. Milk storage bags are typically plastic bags with a secure closure. They generally also have measuring indicators on them so you know how much milk is stored in the bag. It's recommended to only put enough for one bottle in a milk storage bag. This proves helpful if you are planning to be apart from baby because you can give the caretaker the number of bags they'll need for the duration of time they'll be in charge of baby. It takes the guesswork out of making a bottle.

When it comes to bottles, you will likely only need a couple if you're planning to exclusively breastfeed. One thing I found was I had no idea what kind of bottle my baby would prefer. I would recommend ensuring your breastfeeding relationship is well established and baby is comfortable at the breast before introducing a bottle. Then, have a couple of different types of bottles (and nipples) on hand to try out with baby. You can see which bottle baby prefers before buying several more to have on hand.

Another tool I found incredibly helpful was milk collection cups. These are hard plastic shells that sit against your nipple (usually held in place by a bra or tank top). Especially in the early days, I used these in place of breast pads while I was at home. The breast pads are great if you're out and about, but when I was home, I didn't want that liquid gold going to waste! If the idea of wearing them around the house isn't comfortable or it doesn't appeal to you, you can use these while feeding baby. I placed the cup on the nipple baby was not feeding from, and when I had my letdown, the cup collected any milk I leaked. I could then place this milk in a storage bag. Once you and baby establish the breastfeeding relationship and your milk supply levels out, you may find that you don't need to milk collection cups as often. But they're still great to have on hand.

Nipple cream may come in handy, especially in the beginning. Generally speaking, breastfeeding shouldn't be extremely painful unless something is wrong, but that doesn't mean your nipples won't be tender or sore at some point. Nipple creams can help alleviate some of that tenderness that happens in the early days of breastfeeding as your baby acclimates to the breast and your body gets used to breastfeeding.

Another comfort item that might have a dual purpose is a pregnancy pillow. If you find it difficult to get comfortable sleeping while you're pregnant, they have full-body pillows that can help. Once you give birth, that pregnancy pillow can be used to support you and baby while you're breastfeeding. Because baby needs to be held and supported close to the breast if you're in a sitting position, you may find a pillow helpful in holding and supporting your baby. I remember some of the night feeds being difficult because I was just so tired right after my third baby was born, so a pillow helped support her while allowing me to relax a bit more. Anytime you can use something to help you relax and feel more comfortable, you're encouraging your body to make breastfeeding easier. Remember when we discussed the letdown reflex? If you're tense or stressed, your body will have to fight harder for the letdown reflex. A supportive pillow will help alleviate some of the stress and tension that can come with posture while breastfeeding.

You may read (or be told) that you don't *need* anything to successfully breastfeed apart from your body. While that is technically true, your comfort plays an important role in establishing and maintaining a successful breastfeeding relationship. For the most part, the tools and accessories mentioned in this chapter are not necessities, but they'll help you as you navigate and establish your breastfeeding routine with your baby.

CHAPTER 4:

Your First Connection

—◆—

During the first week or so, postpartum can be wonderfully euphoric, celebrating the safe delivery of your perfect baby. However, it can also be stressful as you and baby adjust to a new normal. During this time, focus on your and baby's comfort as you work to establish a successful breastfeeding relationship.

Latching On and Initial Challenges

In the first few hours and days postpartum, it's imperative to work on establishing a correct latch with your baby. Latching onto the breast may seem like an innate skill your baby should possess as it's essential for their survival, but baby will often need some guidance and correction as they navigate their initial feeding sessions. If your baby is unable to successfully latch while nursing, this will result in painful feeding sessions for you and an inadequate removal of milk from the breast, which can lead to a drop in your milk supply and concerns about baby gaining weight.

Before you begin feeding your baby, make sure you're in a comfortable sitting position and your back is supported. When you first feed your baby, focus on supporting baby's head and body and bringing baby to your breast. Hunching over and bringing your breast to baby's mouth will result in poor posture, which will lead to discomfort while you're feeding them. A nursing or pregnancy pillow can assist with supporting baby's body so you can focus on angling and supporting their head correctly.

Before you bring baby to the breast, take the hand not supporting baby's head and make a C shape (as though you're holding a sandwich). Bring your hand to your breast and place your thumb on the top of your breast, above your nipple, just on the edge of your areola. Place your index finger in a similar position on the bottom of your breast. Once you place your fingers, compress your hand slightly to flatten your breast to make it an easier shape for your baby to fit into their mouth. Bring your baby's head toward your breast and trail your nipple along their cheek to initiate the rooting reflex (a reflex in which a baby turns their head looking for a nipple to feed from). Once baby has responded to your touch, position their mouth in front of your nipple and point your nipple toward their nose. Once baby's mouth is open wide, bring your nipple down into their mouth. When baby's mouth closes around the breast, their chin and the tip of their nose should be touching the breast. Their lips should also be flared out on your breast and not tucked or rolled under.

In the early days, your breasts and nipples may be tender or sore as baby works to establish the correct latch. This is normal, and the nipple creams we discussed in the previous chapter can help to alleviate any discomfort. Beyond discomfort or tenderness, prolonged pain can be an indication of an underlying problem. If you notice extreme pain or cracked or bleeding nipples, seek support to determine what the problem might be.

Breastfeeding support groups can also provide physical and emotional support for new moms as they navigate the nuances of motherhood. The La Leche League is an international organization that provides guidance and resources for breastfeeding moms at all stages. After the birth of my first baby, my son, the midwives were invaluable with the help and support they gave me in the hospital to achieve a good latch. I had also attended an antenatal class, and a group of us would regularly meet up post-birth to support each other and voice concerns. Oftentimes, as new moms, we just need to hear that we're doing a great job and everything we're experiencing is normal!

Colostrum and Milk Transition

As mentioned earlier, when you become pregnant, your body will begin to make colostrum, which is a densely nutritious form of breast milk available in the early days. It's thicker than regular breast milk and is more yellow in color. Colostrum is packed with nutrients and antibodies to help build baby's immune system and gut health. It's like a concentrated form of breast milk! Colostrum is easy to digest for your baby (who's been used to receiving their nutrients directly through the umbilical cord) and acts as a laxative to help your baby pass their first bowel movement.

Once your baby is born and your body goes into overdrive to produce milk for your newborn, you'll undoubtedly notice when your milk transitions from colostrum to regular breast milk. For the first week postpartum, your body will contain what is known as transitional milk. As your body works to produce mature breastmilk, your milk will contain traces of colostrum. When your body begins making regular breast milk, this is known as your milk coming in.

In the first few days after your baby is born, you might worry that they're not getting enough to eat because they need to feed so frequently (generally around every three hours). It isn't necessarily that they aren't getting enough to eat; it's more due to the capacity of their stomach. When your baby is born, their stomach is only about as large as a marble and can only accommodate one to two teaspoons of liquid. So naturally, they're going to eat more frequently as their body processes this small amount of food. It isn't until about day ten that your baby's stomach grows in size. About a week and a half following their birth, their stomach will roughly double to about the size of a ping pong ball and be able to hold two ounces of liquid. This might help you understand why newborns seem to eat so frequently! Around one month old, the baby's stomach will grow to be the size of a large egg, and they will be able to ingest anywhere from two and a half to five ounces of liquid.

As your milk matures and baby's stomach grows, you'll find a rhythm to your breastfeeding relationship. Enjoy the first couple of weeks following birth, and allow yourself to focus on what you and baby need as you work together to establish your breastfeeding relationship.

Emotional Adjustments and Baby's Cues

As soon as baby is born, your body begins to undergo many changes. Your hormone levels change, and your body begins healing from birth. You may find yourself overwhelmed and riddled with a myriad of emotions. Between the major life changes and hormonal changes of bringing a baby into the world, it's completely understandable! You'll probably be more emotional, and that's okay. The influx and variation of emotions postpartum is often referred to as baby blues. As your hormones level out, the extreme emotions should as well. However, if you notice it continuing beyond a week or two postpartum, consider speaking to your doctor. If you've ever flown in a plane, you likely know that the flight attendants instruct, in the event of an emergency, to place the oxygen mask on yourself before placing one on your children. Caring for your emotional and mental health is as important as caring for your baby's physical and emotional well-being. Have grace and patience with yourself, and don't be afraid to ask for help if you need it.

As you get to know your baby, you may notice some cues from your baby that indicate they're hungry. Some people assume that a baby cries when they're hungry, but that usually only happens when other more subtle cues have gone unnoticed. You may see your baby smacking their lips or making sucking noises with their mouth. They may also clench their firsts and bring their hands to their mouth to suck on their fists. Another indication of hunger is them moving their head back and forth. This is part of the rooting reflex and is indicative of them looking for the nipple. If you're unable to tend to them with these cues and they escalate to crying, you'll want to soothe them to calm them down before attempting to breastfeed them.

Exploring Breastfeeding Positions and Diaper Changes

Part of getting comfortable with breastfeeding is finding what works for you. In the first week postpartum, you may find your abdomen tender as you heal. Or you may have had a C-section, in which case setting a ten-pound weight above the incision doesn't sound appealing at all! So, let's take a look at some alternatives you can explore and hopefully find your new favorite breastfeeding position!

Traditional Cradle

The traditional cradle hold is one most moms will most likely naturally use because it's simply cradling your baby with one arm, allowing your free hand to manipulate the breast for them if need be. With the cradle hold, you hold the baby with the arm on the side of the body they're breastfeeding from. For example, if baby is nursing from the right breast, you're supporting their body with your right arm, and their head is in the crook of your elbow. If you're breastfeeding twins, the cradle hold can be used to cradle a baby in each arm as they nurse.

Cross Cradle

The cross-cradle hold is similar to the traditional cradle hold. The difference is in how you cradle the baby. In this position, you're using the opposite hand to support them. Begin by holding your baby tummy to tummy with you, with their head positioned in front of the breast they'll be feeding from. If they're feeding from the right breast, use your left hand to hold and position their head. It works best if you place your thumb on the left side of their face, at about their jaw. Then, wrap your hand around the right side of their face, using your middle finger to support their head on their jaw on the other side. Then, with your right hand, you can manipulate your breast for them as needed. Some moms find this position gives them better control and allows them to see what is going on with baby's latch.

Football Hold

In this position, you're going to be placing baby along your side instead of across the front of your body. As the name suggests, you're going to tuck baby under your arm like one might do with a football. So if you're feeding baby on the left side, position baby's body along your left side, positioning their head in front of your breast. This position might be more comfortable with a supporting pillow of some sort. To guide and support baby's head, you'll use your left hand in a similar way to the cross-cradle head. You can then use your right hand to manipulate your breast as needed to get baby to latch on. The football hold works really well for women recovering from a cesarean section (C-section) or for women with larger breasts. For women breastfeeding twins, the football hold works well because you can place a baby on each side of you.

Laid-Back Position

As my babies got older and bigger, we found the lying positions to be an ideal way to nurse, especially first thing in the morning, bedtime, and nighttime feeds.

For this, you partially recline to about a 45-degree angle. This can be achieved by simply laying back on your bed with a pillow supporting you or reclining on a couch.

As you're reclining, lay baby face down along your body so they mimic your position. Place their head at your breast with their torso and legs lying down the front of your body. Baby's hands will generally naturally come up to hug you around the middle or on the breast they're feeding from. This position is great because it allows you a moment to relax and enjoy the moment with your baby.

Side Lying

Side lying is the other position I came to love. In this one, you're going to lie on the side you want baby to feed from, as the name implies. Place baby on their side so they're facing you, trying to get tummy to tummy with them. Some moms find this position easier if they latch the baby sitting up, then they lower down into the side-lying position. Once you get the hang of it, you'll be able to latch baby while lying down with ease! Again, this is a position in which you're able to relax further while baby nurses.

Once you get the hang of different nursing positions and find one(s) that work best for you, you can then use baby's diaper output to help inform you of baby's health. When baby is first born, the colostrum they take in helps them to expel their first bowel movement. Their first bowel movement will be a thick, tar-like substance called meconium. This is perfectly normal and nothing to be alarmed by! As their body expels the meconium, their bowel movements will become more yellow-green in color. Once your milk supply is established and baby has passed all their meconium, you can expect their bowel movements to be yellow or tan in color with a loose, seedy texture. Sometimes, what you eat can affect the color of their bowel movements, but for the most part, color, texture, and number of bowel movements can be a good way to inform you if something is going on with baby.

Remember, the first week postpartum is all about getting to know your baby and establishing the foundation for a lifelong connection. Focus on comfort and what works for your dyad. Establish a successful latch with baby, find positions that work to keep you and baby at ease, and get in tune with your baby's body and cues.

CHAPTER 5:

The Breastfeeding Diet

—◆—

As you adjust to life with a newborn baby, a balanced diet may be the furthest thing from your mind. But it's important to take care of your needs nutritionally, not only to nourish your body for yourself but because your body takes what you put in to produce your breast milk. Let's take a look at some tips and concerns that may come up.

Nourishing Yourself for Breastfeeding

When preparing meals for yourself while breastfeeding, a balanced, healthy diet is important. It's also a good idea to follow dietary guidelines from when you were pregnant. For example, you still want to limit the consumption of fish that contains high levels of mercury. But aside from that, focus on incorporating a variety of foods. It's recommended to have seven and a half servings of vegetables and legumes a day and nine servings of grains a day. This might seem like a lot! But if you make sure to include at least one to two servings in each meal, you can always have snacks throughout the day that include vegetables, legumes, and grains. Then it's recommended to get two servings of fruits, two and a half servings of a source of protein, and two and a half servings of dairy or a dairy alternative. If this feels overwhelming, try not to focus on the numbers. Just remember that you need vegetables, legumes, and grains the most. Variety will ensure you get the nutrients you need without having to feel like you need to keep track of them constantly.

Food Safety and Practicality

As you prepare your food at home and may occasionally go out to eat, be mindful of proper food handling. Eating undercooked food puts you at risk for foodborne illnesses. This can lead to possible food poisoning, which can leave you incapacitated. Breastfeeding your baby may become incredibly challenging if you're struck with an ailment from not properly preparing food. Ensure your meats are cooked to the correct temperature and foods are stored correctly to avoid any concerns with contamination after they are cooked. In addition to mercury being a concern from certain fish, eating raw fish may best be avoided until you are no longer breastfeeding your baby.

Vitamins, Caloric Needs, and Special Considerations

It is often recommended that breastfeeding women take vitamin supplements while breastfeeding. Some healthcare providers may recommend breastfeeding moms continue taking their prenatal vitamins. Vitamin D is also often recommended as a supplement for breastfeeding women to take, but check with your doctor first for peace of mind. For example, I consume a drink that helps alleviate symptoms of IBS. The product is made from all-natural ingredients and is advertised as safe while breastfeeding, but I still checked with my doctor beforehand to ensure it was safe to drink while I was breastfeeding.

In addition to knowing about potential supplements, it's also important to realize that making breast milk burns extra calories. You'll need about 300–500 additional calories to account for the extra work your body is doing. As mentioned above, a balanced diet is important, but don't feel bad about indulging in a slice of cake every now and then.

Something I wasn't aware of before breastfeeding was an unquenchable thirst! It's imperative to keep yourself hydrated as well as nourished. You don't need to go crazy with water consumption, but make sure you're listening to your body and drinking to quell your thirst. I found that I would feel incredibly thirsty just before my letdown reflex kicked in. I made sure to always have water available while I was breastfeeding. Some women will have a specific breastfeeding area set up in their home, where they ensure they always have water, a comfortable place to nurse, and reading material or something to do while nursing. Some women also find that having a warm beverage while nursing helps with their letdown reflex. I found that I needed water before anything else.

Listening to your body and taking care of your needs will ensure that you're prepared to care for baby in all ways.

Managing Caffeine and Alcohol

When it comes to indulgences like caffeine and alcohol, moderation is key. It's not necessary to completely avoid either. Being a new mom adjusting to the schedule and demands of a newborn baby, you're likely going to be tired and reach for caffeine. This is understandable and perfectly okay! If you do reach for caffeine, just be mindful of when and how often. If you can, consume caffeine shortly following a nursing session, as by the next time you nurse baby, there will be fewer traces of caffeine in your breast milk. Caffeine can transfer to breast milk, so if you have more than usual, you may notice baby's sleep patterns being affected. It's worth noting that caffeine isn't only present in coffee. If you regularly drink coffee, be aware of other things you might eat or drink that contain caffeine as well. For example, chocolate contains caffeine as well as soda. So, if you want to indulge in one of the aforementioned things, consider limiting your coffee intake to avoid overwhelming your system with caffeine.

Alcohol maintains a similar principle to caffeine. It's recommended that if you're going to consume alcohol, wait at least two hours before breastfeeding. Having a drink occasionally won't have any negative effects on your baby. But if you overindulge, not only are you risking passing alcohol to your baby through the breast milk, but breastfeeding while under the influence of alcohol can be dangerous for baby. You want to make sure you're alert while breastfeeding and excessive alcohol consumption can definitely impair that.

Being a mom doesn't mean not being able to enjoy the things you used to before you became pregnant. It just means being mindful of the impact those things have on your baby.

From Mother to Baby

As mentioned in the last chapter, a baby's bowel movements can be an indication of something going on with baby's body. Sometimes, it might be an alert of an illness, or it could just be baby reacting to something you ate or drank. Remember, a food log can come in handy in the early days. If you notice baby displaying discomfort possibly from a tummy ache, or they have an explosive diaper, you can reference your food log to determine if something you ate triggered the reaction. For example, when I was breastfeeding my daughter, she would struggle the day after I ate curry. But now it's one of her favorite foods! A sensitivity or reaction doesn't indicate a lifetime aversion. Sometimes, their little tummies are just sensitive to new spices or textures.

Being attentive to your baby's needs and reactions can go a long way in making both of you comfortable and at ease!

CHAPTER 6:

Comfort and Convenience

—◆—

In chapter three, we discussed nursing bras and maternity clothes serving dual purposes, but in this chapter, we're going to dive a bit deeper into what kind of wardrobe can contribute to a positive breastfeeding experience.

Choosing the Right Nursing Bras

As discussed previously, nursing bras will become an essential part of your breastfeeding wardrobe. There are a multitude of styles to choose from. It's just a matter of finding what's most comfortable and accessible for you. Bandeau nursing bras are typically made of a breathable material that pulls on over your head. They lack a clasp at the back, which may be more comfortable. They do have clasps on the front straps that serve to release the material from the bra to expose the breast. Additionally, the soft structure can keep your breasts from escaping the confines of the bra. The main downside with this type of bra is the potential lack of support, especially in the early days when your breasts might be larger than normal and may become engorged between feedings.

V-neck seamless bras are another option that lacks a clasp in the back. The difference with this type is that instead of having a clasp to release the material, the bra is designed with a V to allow you to move the material aside easily to expose the breast. This type of bra is comfortable for the same reason the bandeau bra is. In addition to that, you can wear a V-neck top with this type of bra and not have to worry about exposing your bra. However, because the material moves aside with ease, this can contribute to your boobs more easily escaping, creating the dreaded third and fourth boobs! Escaping nipples can also be a concern. If you're still experiencing leaking, this can present a problem because your breast pad would remain in the bra while the leaking nipple has escaped. This may result in a dampened shirt, requiring an impromptu outfit change.

I do realize that every woman is different, so this may not be your experience! That's why it's important to try different styles to find what might suit you best.

Non-wired, traditionally shaped nursing bras have a clasp at the back like a normal bra. In addition, they have claps at the front on the straps that release the cup so you can easily breastfeed. These types of bras are likely to be less comfortable than a bandeau bra or the V-neck seamless bra. But they do provide more support and structure. These may work best for when you need to leave the house or want more support in your bra. I've collected several different styles that I use as a need arises.

Wired traditional-style nursing bras are also available, and they have a similar structure to the bras mentioned previously. They include an underwire in the front of the bra. I found these to be uncomfortable, and if you can avoid wired bras, it is better. The wire of the bra can dig into your breast tissue and affect your milk supply and output.

Whichever option appeals to you, focus on that which will be comfortable and encourage you to easily breastfeed your baby without much fuss.

Creating a Nursing-Friendly Wardrobe

As mentioned previously, you may be able to continue to wear pregnancy clothes throughout postpartum. You can also find clothes specifically designed to make breastfeeding easier. But it's not entirely necessary to purchase an entirely new wardrobe for breastfeeding. Button-down shirts, cardigans, and V-neck tops can prove to be incredibly effective while breastfeeding and can often be found in your closet from before you became pregnant.

If you have to attend a special event, it can be overwhelming trying to plan an outfit. Breastfeeding-friendly clothes are available, but you can also use regular clothes. If you don't want to have to purchase dresses or outfits designed specifically for breastfeeding, look for V-neck tops with stretch material that can easily be moved aside to access the breast. Additionally, tops with thin straps can serve well by allowing you to pull the strap down.

Something to keep in mind as you look for an outfit, whether for daily wear or a special occasion, consider the material the clothing is made of. Is it something that can be easily washed if breast milk or spit-up gets on it? For example, silk may not be your best friend when it comes to your breastfeeding options.

When it comes to your clothes, keep function and comfort at the forefront of your mind. Ask yourself if the article of clothing will allow you to breastfeed your baby with ease and if it will be able to be easily cleaned in the event of leaking or spills.

Layering It On

One thing I found that was the most helpful while breastfeeding was wearing layers. Layers not only allow for easy feeding but they can also contribute to discreet feeding. I typically wore a tank top underneath a T-shirt or sweater. If baby became hungry in public, I was able to lift the top layer to expose my breast while being able to keep my stomach covered up. The top shirt also served to cover part of my exposed breast. Despite knowing I shouldn't have to feel self-conscious while nursing my baby (whether in public or in private), it allowed me to feel like there was less of a chance of flashing my boob at a passerby. Additionally, as baby gets older, they're more likely to be curious. While they're feeding, they may pop off the breast to look around, in which case you can easily lower your shirt until they return to breastfeeding.

Scarves and shawls can also be quite useful in the layering process. They serve to be an accessory or to keep you warm as a wardrobe choice. But in the event that your baby is easily distracted, the scarf or shawl can be used to drape over your shoulder to cover baby as they're breastfeeding. This may keep them from being distracted by sights and sounds around them. But be warned, some babies may not mind having a thin cloth draped over them, while other babies may prove to hate it. Again, it's about finding what works for you and baby and supports your breastfeeding goals.

Your wardrobe may be one of the last things you consider as you're preparing to breastfeed, but having clothes that make breastfeeding easier can go a long way in taking some of the stress out of nursing.

CHAPTER 7:

Partners in the Night

—◆—

We all know sleep is important for our bodies. Experts recommend adults get between seven and eight hours of sleep at night, and often, this is manageable... without children. Once you have a newborn baby, you may find yourself trying to negotiate with the universe for sleep. Below, we'll explore why sleep is important and how you can ensure you and baby are getting enough—no negotiating with the universe required.

The Importance of Sleep for Parents and Babies

With proper sleep, our bodies are healthier, our memories are sharper, and we feel better overall. This applies to babies and adults. When babies sleep, their bodies produce a protein that assists their body when they're under the weather. So not only is it important for them to get proper sleep at night, but if they do get sick, you might notice they sleep more. Let them! It's their body's first line of natural defense. In addition to working to improve their immune system, a baby's body releases a growth hormone that contributes to their physical development. So those hours of sleep at night help them grow strong as well as healthy!

Have you ever had a rough night's sleep or simply didn't get enough? You probably weren't all that pleasant to be around because the lack of sleep made you more irritable and crankier. This can happen to babies as well. Sometimes, if they're more fussy than normal or they're harder to calm down, it may be because they didn't get enough sleep or adequate sleep the night before. If that happens, give them some extra love and care and try to get them to take an extra nap so they can get the rest they need.

This brings me to the importance of sleep for moms. As mentioned, when we don't sleep well, it can impact the following day in negative ways. Not only are we likely to be easier to anger, but we also may have brain fog and won't be as sharp as we normally would be. When you have a newborn, getting adequate sleep for you is just as important as it is for baby. If you're being plagued by exhaustion, it can negatively impact how you respond to your baby or reduce your response time because you're not as alert. Exhaustion can also heighten depression and anxiety. Earlier, we talked about baby blues as your hormones level out. Getting enough sleep is important to assist your body in leveling out these hormones so we don't exacerbate the effect of those baby blues. To ensure you're strengthening your connection with your baby as much as you can, prioritize your sleep in the early weeks at home with baby.

When I say prioritize your sleep, I don't mean neglecting baby's need for nighttime feedings. As we discussed previously, nighttime feeds are incredibly important for baby. A newborn has no concept of night and day. The only thing they know is to alert someone when their body displays signs of discomfort, such as when they're hungry. It's a good idea to adjust your sleep to your baby's instead of trying to adjust your baby's sleep to yours. As you work to meet their needs in the first few weeks, they'll get more used to the difference between night and day, and will likely start staying awake longer during the day, resulting in eventually sleeping longer at night.

The first few weeks postpartum can be particularly difficult as you adjust to your newborn's evolving sleep patterns. One thing that might help is establishing a nighttime routine. This will help baby get used to cues that indicate it's time to wind down, but it will also help you train your body to go to sleep when baby does. If you're used to being a night owl or going to bed later, this might be a challenge for you. But going to bed a little bit earlier might help you get better sleep even if you're waking up with baby several times throughout the night. Some things you can do to establish a nighttime routine are giving baby a bath (the warm water helps relax them), making sure the lights in the house are dim, and reading a book to baby. If you do this every night, baby will soon recognize these as signs that it's time for them to get ready for sleep. It also helps to put baby down for the night when they're sleepy. Doing a nighttime routine can help relax them and make them more tired, making it easier to put them down to sleep. If they're awake and alert, they may just fuss when you put them down and likely won't be any closer to sleep just because they're in a dark room.

Exploring Sleep Solutions

Despite the numerous books by "experts," most new mothers will struggle with bringing baby home and getting adequate sleep in those first few weeks. The often-given advice "sleep when baby sleeps" does have some merit, though. As mentioned above, try and get into the habit of going to sleep when you put baby down for the night and during the day; if you're finding yourself exhausted, take advantage of baby napping during the day and allow yourself a nap as well. It may not always be feasible, but getting enough rest is more important than switching out that load of laundry or putting away the clean dishes. The dishes and laundry can be handled when you have a chance to rest and recharge. But if you attempt to manage household tasks instead of getting some sleep, you're just putting yourself at more of a disadvantage to be able to care for baby and yourself. A well-rested momma is a happy momma!

If you have a partner, consider asking them to help out if possible. This may mean that the division of chores in the house shifts while you acclimate to your baby's needs. If your partner is able to, have them help at night as well. For example, at night, if you wake up to feed the baby and notice they need a diaper change, you can ask your partner to handle the nonfeeding tasks during the night or have them help settle baby back to sleep after they've fed. If your partner has to work, this may not be as feasible. But if you're struggling to get good sleep at night, talk to your partner and see if you can come up with ways they can help you so you can make sure you're getting the rest you need.

Additionally, consider your sleeping arrangements. When my babies were newborns and waking several times throughout the night, I opted to have a bassinet in my bedroom. This allowed me to wake more easily but not have to wake fully by trudging to another room to feed them. Co-sleeping is common in some cultures, but some experts are divided on it. Especially in the early days when you're exhausted, co-sleeping may not be as safe (because you don't wake up as easily at night).

Talk to your partner and discuss different solutions you can try out that will contribute to a restful night for you and baby! Many people will try and tell you what you should (or shouldn't) be doing or what they did, but you need to focus on doing what's right (and best) for you and your family. The well-intended advice from outsiders sounds well and good when they give it, but they aren't the ones battling exhaustion.

Navigating Changing Sleep Patterns

Remember that for nine months, your baby was in a climate-controlled environment and they had no concept of night and day. In fact, it's not uncommon for babies to be more active in utero during the night. This is because, during the day, your movements are essentially rocking them and soothing them. Once you stop moving and settle down for the night, they don't have those same soothing motions. As babies become familiar with your routines, it will help them acclimate to the world outside the womb. This is where those nighttime routines can come in handy.

Typically, newborn babies are going to sleep quite a bit and won't differentiate between night and day. As they get older, you'll notice that they sleep less and less. The goal is to get them to get most of their sleep in at night and be awake and alert during the day. But this will take time.

It's not uncommon for new parents to get a slew of visits when they have a newborn. Everyone is so excited to meet your baby! And while you may want to accommodate visitors, don't be afraid to say no. Especially if they want to visit in the evening and potentially interrupt the nighttime routine you're trying to establish. They can visit you and baby once you've had more time to get used to baby and their evolving sleep patterns.

One thing to keep in mind is to teach baby that nighttime is for sleeping. Yes, they'll wake up for their night feedings, but when that happens, don't turn on all the lights and talk to them in a normal speaking voice. If you have to get out of bed to feed them, turn on as few lights as possible so they don't think the light is signaling it's time to sleep. Also, try to respond to their hunger cues at night as quickly as possible. The more baby works themself up, the harder they'll be to settle back down to go to sleep. Soon, your baby will be able to tell the difference between day and night feeds, and they'll be easier to put back to sleep during nighttime feedings.

It can be incredibly frustrating, but as cliche as it sounds, remind yourself that it won't last. By about three months, babies start to sleep longer stretches throughout the night. So the sleepless nights won't be happening forever. Have grace with yourself and your baby. Some nights, it might feel like your baby was sent to test your sanity. But remind yourself that you're their frame of reference. They have no idea how the world works, so it's your job to model healthy sleep patterns and soothe them when they hit a rough patch.

It also bears importance to note that there will be factors beyond your control that can impact their sleep. For example, if they're under the weather or have a tummy ache, they may have a harder time settling down to go to sleep. Other things like teething and growth spurts can also impact their sleep. So if you've established a great sleep routine and it seems like your baby is sleeping more at night, only for them to suddenly be waking more at night, stay calm. Continue to keep night feedings quiet and stick to your nighttime routines. It won't always be perfect, but that familiarity can also provide baby comfort in stretches where their sleep patterns are being interrupted.

In the first few weeks postpartum, make your and baby's health and well-being a priority. This means ensuring you're both getting enough sleep and working to establish a healthy breastfeeding relationship. You won't get a do-over of those early weeks, so make them count!

CHAPTER 8:

Liquid Gold

—◆—

Mother's breast milk is a complete nutritional meal for your baby if they're exclusively breastfeeding. If you don't work outside the home, you may not see a need to consider expressing milk. But as we discussed earlier, there can be a myriad of reasons why you may want to express milk besides having to work outside the home.

The Benefits and Options of Expressing Milk

In the early days, before I went back to work, I found myself sometimes needing to express milk to relieve my engorged breasts when my milk first came in, as well as while my supply evened out. I also found it helpful to pump milk to build a stash so that if I wanted to go out for the evening, I wouldn't have to worry about getting back in time to be able to feed my baby. A benefit to building a stash is that when I started to introduce my baby to solids, I was able to mix different foods with my breast milk, so I was introducing a new flavor or texture with something he was familiar with.

If you're not planning to work full-time once baby is older, you may be asking why you would even need to consider pumping. As mentioned above, it helps to have breast milk on hand in case you need to be away from baby. Having breast milk on hand gives you the option to have a date night with your spouse, enjoy a night out with friends, or just have an extended trip to the store without having to rush back to feed baby. Additionally, your partner may want to be involved in feeding baby, and that can be difficult if you're exclusively feeding from the breast. Bottle-feeding breast milk allows your partner to experience feeding the baby and gives them an opportunity to get comfortable with baby's cues if they need to feed them when you're not around.

Choosing the Right Equipment

There are a multitude of breast pumps available. I felt like manual pumps were effective if I wanted to pump to relieve engorgement or if I just wanted to collect a small amount. But if I needed to pump for an extended period, using a mechanical pump was easier and less work for me.

As with most products, automatic breast pumps range from basic and affordable to expensive with all the bells and whistles. Generally, a basic breast pump will get the job done just fine. If you're in the United States, it may be worth contacting your insurance, as some insurances provide you with a breast pump. They may send you a breast pump, or you might have to purchase one and they reimburse you up to a certain amount. Either way, it's definitely worth looking into!

Choosing a pump depends on what you will need it for. If you will be staying home with baby, a manual pump may be just fine or a basic electric pump. But if you're going back to work, you may find an electric pump to be more useful.

Something I discovered with my daughter, my third child, was milk collection cups. These are small, hard plastic shells that are worn inside the bra. These are handy if you're breastfeeding because you can place them on the breast baby isn't feeding from and collect any milk that leaks. This is a great way to preserve your liquid gold instead of it being absorbed by a breast pad.

Wearable breast pumps can be worn inside the bra, providing a more discreet option for pumping. These are great options for a quick session to relieve engorgement or if you're in a pinch and need to pump. Discreet pumps are also helpful while baby is nursing. Not only can the pump collect milk from your letdown, but it can also encourage more milk, so if you're trying to build a stash, you won't have to work as hard.

For a mom who has to work full-time and pump for baby, discreet or wearable pumps may not be as practical. Moms who are pumping most of the day may find a full-size mechanical breast pump works best and can keep up with the amount of pumping they need to do.

Expressed Milk for Bottle Feeding and Storage

Once you collect breast milk either from pumping or utilizing collection cups while breastfeeding, now what?

We previously discussed milk storage bags. These are an easy and effective way of storing your breast milk, and it can be helpful to know how much is in the bag. When I would pump, I would pour my milk into the collection bag and write the date and time on the bag as well as how many ounces it was. I did this because I would store the bags in the freezer lying flat. In that position, I wouldn't be able to know just by looking at it how many ounces were in it. The time is helpful to note because if you're a coffee drinker, trace amounts of caffeine may be more prevalent in your milk in the earlier hours of the day. In this case, you wouldn't want your baby to be given a bottle of that breast milk. Additionally, breast milk made and pumped at night typically has higher levels of sleep hormones. So you would want to note any milk you've pumped at night in case your baby needs a nighttime bottle, as this may be the better option to give them.

Fresh breast milk can be stored in the refrigerator for up to four days. If you don't plan on using the breast milk right away, place it in the freezer. Breast milk can be stored frozen for up to six months. Once you pull breast milk out to thaw and serve to your baby, it's not recommended to freeze it again. This is why I would only place as much milk in one storage bag that baby would need per bottle. Any milk not used that has been defrosted can be kept in the fridge for up to twenty-four hours. And in the off-chance that baby doesn't finish their bottle, the bottle can be placed in the fridge for two hours, but it's not recommended to serve milk beyond that timeframe to a baby.

But what happens to your frozen milk stash in the event of a power outage? In my first experience with this, I panicked. I was so afraid I was going to have to throw away all my liquid gold and rebuild my stash.

However, I learned that if your breast milk has begun to thaw but still has frozen crystals in it, it is safe to freeze it. Only if the milk is completely thawed do you have to use it within twenty-four hours. So, if you lose power or even take out an extra bag of milk, check to see if it still has milk crystals in it. If it does, you can safely place it back in the freezer.

If you find that you have breast milk in the freezer beyond the six-month mark or you have milk that you defrosted but didn't use, don't throw it out! Some people will use the breast milk that they can't feed to baby in bath water, especially if baby has sensitive skin. Or you can draw up your own milk bath!

Challenges With Expressed Milk

As with breastfeeding, expressing milk comes with its own set of challenges. If you're not away from baby, it can be an inconvenience to have to pump in addition to breastfeeding. Some women may feel like they constantly have something attached to their boob in the first few months postpartum if they're exclusively breastfeeding as well as trying to build up a stash.

If you find expressing to be stressful, don't do it! Once again, do what works best for you and baby. Some people find they don't have time to pump, which was the case with my third child. I generally had some milk in the freezer in the event that I had to be away from her, but I also had a couple of bottles worth of formula available in the event that she needed to be fed while I was away and there wasn't enough breast milk available.

Balancing getting to know your baby, establishing a breastfeeding relationship, and ensuring you and baby are getting enough rest is a lot of work! So if not expressing is a relief to you, don't feel guilty about it. On the other hand, if expressing your milk brings you satisfaction, that is okay too! Some women aren't able to feed baby from the breast, and being able to provide breast milk through expressing can be gratifying. The goal is to meet your baby's basic needs, however that looks for you. There isn't any judgment in making decisions for you and baby that support your health and well-being.

CHAPTER 9:

Getting Out and About

—◆—

When you and baby first get home after leaving the hospital, leaving the house might be the furthest thing from your mind. As we mentioned previously, in the first couple of weeks, you probably just want to focus on getting adequate rest and establishing your breastfeeding relationship. But after those first few weeks, you'll find yourself getting into a routine and rhythm as you tune into baby's needs and cues. Once you get there, leaving the house won't be so daunting.

The Importance of Going Out

Whether we're introverts or extroverts, staying cooped up in the house all the time might lead us to feel stir-crazy. If you're feeling anxious or antsy but you're getting adequate rest and taking care of your physical needs, maybe it's time to step outside! Whether it's for a quick stroll around the block, just to run errands, or even to socialize with friends, it's important to venture out of the confines of the house every now and again. Exposing yourself to fresh air and sun can have a positive impact on your mental health.

Humans crave connection. It's part of our subconscious need. We need interactions with others to thrive. In the first few weeks postpartum, most of your interactions will likely be with your baby and your partner (and any other family you might have at home). But stepping out of the house exposes you to the other people. If you're running to the grocery store really quick, you likely won't have any life-changing conversations, but just being surrounded by other people can bring a sense of calm and normality to your life.

Being at home with your baby in the beginning can feel natural and easy. But it can also feel isolating. Meeting with a friend for coffee can help you take in some fresh air and human connection. If you're not quite ready to brave an outing with baby, consider just taking a walk around your neighborhood. You'll likely run into neighbors who will be excited to see you and baby.

Additionally, going for a walk outside is great for your and baby's health. Some babies need vitamin D supplements because Mom isn't getting enough and there are only trace amounts in their breast milk. But taking a 15- to 30-minute walk outside when the sun is shining can allow you and baby to get the vitamin D you need. The fresh air can be rejuvenating, and the sun is literally good for your health!

If getting out of the house in the early weeks seems impossible, take it slow. Maybe you just go outside to check the mail or walk around your yard. Try to work up to being able to be outside for longer periods of time. Getting out of the house and eventually meeting up with a friend can have profound impacts on your mental health. You may not even realize how much you need the human connection until you're in the middle of a conversation. A happy momma leads to a happy baby. Taking care of your mental health is just as important as taking care of your physical health!

Preparing for Outings With Baby

As with most things, preparation can be the difference between a successful or a disastrous outing with baby. Packing a bag ahead of time with everything you need will not only ensure you're ready for any scenario, but it can also help you prepare mentally in case you have any anxiety about going out into public with baby. Oftentimes, the cause of anxiety is our brain cataloging all the "worst-case scenarios." Our mind is working overtime, trying to determine what could possibly go wrong. But what our brain doesn't do is provide solutions for those scenarios. Take that anxiety by the horns and examine those worst-case scenarios; determine your solutions (or things you might need) if any of those things might happen. This can help quell that anxiety and help you feel more confident about the outing, no matter how big or small it is.

Most moms will have a diaper bag prepared with the different things you'll need to change baby's diaper while you're on the go. But having changing supplies is just one thing you need to be prepared for. A change of clothes might be something you add in the event of a messy diaper or an accident while nursing. You might also consider adding a lightweight blanket or two to your bag. Muslin blankets are great because they're thin and don't take up a lot of room. If you pack one or two of those, you can use them to bundle baby up if it gets chilly, or they can also serve as a discreet cover if you breastfeed in public.

When you pack your bag for baby, consider adding a few items in for yourself, too. Being prepared also means considering what you might need while you're out with your baby. In addition to packing a spare outfit for baby, someone told me that I should also pack an outfit change for myself, and that was the best advice I ever received! Accidents happen. Whether leaky nipples or spit-up from baby, you might find yourself in a situation where a soiled shirt ruins the moment for you. Instead of powering through it or contemplating going home, think ahead and pack an extra top for yourself. To avoid making my baby bag too bulky, I didn't pack an entire outfit change for myself, but I made sure I always had an extra top on hand. You also might want to ensure you have a few extra breast pads. If you've established breastfeeding with your baby and your supply has evened out, you may not need extra breast pads. But because they don't take up much room, it doesn't hurt to have them in your bag, just in case!

Preparing to go out with baby can be a little overwhelming as you try to catalog everything you might need. It might help if you have a partner or friend with you when you go out with baby for the first time. A reassuring presence can remind you of what you might need and help ease your nerves. Once you're out with baby, you may realize that you were worried about nothing! But if the outing doesn't go as planned, don't write it off as normal! Also give yourself permission to turn around and go home if it's too overwhelming. Your mental health is of the utmost importance, and you need to listen to your body. If you're stressed and anxious, baby will be able to pick up on that, and it might make them fussy. So, if you made the attempt and you're just not feeling it, do what's best for you and head back home. There's always tomorrow to try again.

There are bound to be some bumps in the road as you get used to accommodating baby in your life when you used to be able to just up and go whenever and wherever you wanted. But if something doesn't go according to plan, remind yourself that it's a learning experience. Determine if there's something you could have done or prepared differently. If so, use that the next time you go out. The more you do it, the easier it will get!

Dealing With Breastfeeding in Public

Depending on who you talk to, breastfeeding in public can be seen as a hot topic. You'll find that some people are incredibly accommodating and see nothing wrong with a mother feeding her baby in public from her breast. Other people will see it as inappropriate and feel as though mothers should only breastfeed in private. The most important thing to note is that you're doing what's natural by breastfeeding your baby, whether you're at home or in public. Most places have laws in place that protect breastfeeding mothers. Unfortunately, the stigma and judgment from people who don't believe breastfeeding mothers have a right to nurse their baby whenever and wherever they want can negatively impact a new mother's confidence in breastfeeding in public.

Some women are the picture of ease as they breastfeed their babies in public. They appear comfortable and completely unbothered. Unfortunately, that wasn't me. When I would nurse my baby in public, I found myself constantly looking around to see if anyone was looking or judging me. I was silently praying my baby would cooperate and stay latched. I was so worried they would unlatch and throw their head back, exposing my breast to anyone passing by. One time, I took my eight-week-old to a public pool with the rest of our family. Before I had a chance to sit down, he started crying, so I discreetly latched him on before getting settled in. I moved to sit on the shaded chaise longue but made a fatal error when I sat on the side of the chair where the head normally goes. No legs supported the head end, so I ended up with the chaise longue flipped over on me, swallowing me whole. My main concern at that moment was my baby. I clutched him to my chest as I had to be pried out of the chair. Once I was free, I checked on my son, only to realize he had unlatched during the ordeal. So now all the extra attention I had drawn went right to my exposed breast. Talk about a mortifying experience!

There really isn't any way to prepare for a horrifying experience like mine. It's one of those things where you just have to shake it off, remind yourself that everyone has breasts, and that you weren't doing anything nefarious. Mishaps are bound to happen, but being able to brush it off is a skill that will go a long way!

One source of anxiety can come when baby gets older. As babies grow and develop, they naturally become more interested in the world around them. This may result in them suddenly unlatching to look around, which might result in you flashing someone unintentionally. Wearing layers in public can help because not only will your midsection be covered, but you can also quickly cover your breast with your top shirt if baby pops off during a nursing session. Muslin blankets are also handy because you can drape them over your shoulder, and since they're lightweight, baby usually isn't bothered by having that over them. Some babies are more particular, though, and they may want to play with the blanket while nursing, especially if they don't want it covering them. You can find specialty nursing covers if you find this is the case with your baby. They have some that are made of lightweight fabric with an arched neckline that keeps the cover away from your body. This allows baby to nurse without something directly on top of them, and it also allows you to see your baby and provide them that stimulation as they get older. So, if you worry about baby popping off the breast and giving someone a show, these may be a great option!

Apprehension about breastfeeding in public is completely normal. But remind yourself that your body was made to nourish your baby, and that's exactly what you're doing. If someone has a problem with you breastfeeding in public, that's *their* problem, not yours. You have every right to be in public breastfeeding your baby, and as mentioned, most places have laws in place that prevent someone from requesting you relocate while nursing your baby.

Just like getting out of the house with baby, breastfeeding in public gets easier the more you do it. Sure, some people might not agree with it, but others will encourage you. I had many women give me words of encouragement when I would breastfeed my baby in public. Those instances of affirmation really helped quell my nerves and remind me that I'm doing the best I can for my baby. I don't need to be weighed down by the judgments or misinformed opinions of others.

Some women discover that no matter how many times they breastfeed in public, it never gets easier. If you find that's the case, do what works for you. You can always express milk ahead of time and have it available to give baby a bottle or use formula if you don't have access to a way to keep the expressed milk cold. Life as a parent comes with a myriad of challenges; make it more manageable by doing what is easier for you. If you find that breastfeeding in public makes you anxious and you don't want to leave the house because of it, take steps to eliminate that hurdle. There is no judgment in how you choose to feed your baby to support your well-being.

CHAPTER 10:

Breastfeeding Hurdles

—◆—

As with most things related to parenthood, you'll inevitably run into some challenges when it comes to breastfeeding. We're going to discuss some of the common issues you might encounter in your breastfeeding relationship and how you can navigate them should they arise.

Mastitis and Other Painful Challenges

Mastitis

One of the things you may experience when you're breastfeeding is mastitis. Mastitis is an infection in the breast that happens when the milk ducts become clogged and aren't cleared. That, combined with the bacteria from baby nursing, can cause an infection in the breast where the clog is located. Mastitis has a higher chance of setting in if the breasts aren't emptied regularly or with short and infrequent feedings. Bacteria can also fester and contribute to mastitis if you have a cracked nipple.

When you first get mastitis, you may notice that your breast is tender or sore, and there may be a localized red area on the skin where the discomfort is. This is then accompanied by a fever and flu-like symptoms. I developed mastitis with my second baby, another son, not realizing the flu-like symptoms were related to my incredibly sore breasts.

You'll typically be able to pinpoint where the clogged milk duct is because it will be warm to the touch, and the tenderness or soreness will be centrally located in one spot. If you're not sure, gently massage around your breast and see if you can identify where it might be originating from.

Mastitis is definitely treatable and can often be resolved at home without a medical care provider. When I got mastitis, I was able to take steps to alleviate my symptoms, and thankfully, I was well within twenty-four hours.

When you notice mastitis setting in, one of the first things you can try and do is have your baby breastfeed. Keeping the milk ducts clear can potentially help dislodge the clod causing the infection. Applying a warm compress or taking a warm shower can help alleviate some of the pain as well as help possibly loosen up the clogged duct. Massage can also help. You can do this while you're in the warm shower so it will be easier to glide along your skin. To massage the clogged milk duct, you first want to identify where it is. Once you're able to get an idea of where the clogged milk duct is, take your fingers and start *behind* the milk duct (closer to your body). Gently massage forward toward the nipple in circular motions. Another tip I discovered from some mom friends is to use a comb. You'll do the same thing as when you massaged the breast; start behind the breast and "comb" toward the nipple. This might work best in the shower or with some nipple cream applied to the breast. Something else you can try that absolutely blew my mind is using an electric toothbrush. If you have an electric toothbrush, turn it on and then (the same as the comb and massage technique) start behind the clog and move forward to the nipple. This unconventional technique is effective because the vibrations from the toothbrush can help in dislodging the clog.

Dangle feeding can also be helpful in dislodging clogged ducts. If you've established a good latch with your baby and you find yourself with mastitis, consider trying this breastfeeding position! To do this, lay baby on the ground and hover above baby. You may start out on your hands and knees, but you may need to crouch lower to bring the breast closer to baby. For this position, it's exactly as it sounds. You're going to breastfeed baby while your breasts are dangling. In this position, gravity can help dislodge a clog by working with the baby's suckling motion.

The mastitis I had with my second son cleared up quickly with the help of my son feeding and massage. Following the birth of my fourth child, another boy, I recently developed mastitis, and this took longer to get under control. My doctor did prescribe antibiotics. However, as soon as I'd collected them, I started to feel better, so I didn't end up taking them.

When you first feel like you have mastitis, consider giving the above tips a try if you are able to. If more than twenty-four hours have passed and your fever persists, consider reaching out to your healthcare provider. If mastitis doesn't resolve on its own, you'll need antibiotics to clear up the infection.

Some women will be fortunate enough to never have to experience mastitis, but others may have the misfortune of struggling with it. It's anybody's guess where you might fall! A friend of mine was determined to breastfeed her son, but unfortunately, she was plagued with mastitis. She got it so often and severely that she ended up developing an abscess, so she made the decision that it wasn't healthy for her to continue to breastfeed. Because of the symptoms, it was making her sick, and she was drained physically, mentally, and emotionally. So, making the decision to discontinue breastfeeding supported her overall well-being. Once she stopped breastfeeding, the mastitis had an opportunity to clear up, and she was like a new woman: happy and healthy. In turn, her son was happy, healthy, and still fed!

Breastfeeding is functional, and while it has some hurdles, it should be enjoyable. You shouldn't have to suffer being unwell and miserable.

Tongue and Lip Ties

My second and fourth babies, both boys, were tongue-tied. It was noticed before leaving the hospital after the birth of my second son. As it was more severe, they booked an appointment for him to have it cut at a few weeks old. With my fourth baby, we only found out he was tongue-tied at around weeks old, but it was very mild, and we were advised to leave it.

If baby is struggling to develop a good latch, you might want to consider having them evaluated for a tie. When a baby is plagued with a tongue or lip tie, they aren't able to latch properly because the skin is restricting the movement of the mouth and tongue. Some doctors might diagnose your baby with a lip tie, but if baby is successfully breastfeeding and isn't demonstrating any concerns such as weight loss and you aren't experiencing pain while breastfeeding, your doctor may not opt to correct the lip tie.

However, tongue and lip ties don't only impact breastfeeding. If your baby has a tie but they don't get diagnosed, it can potentially impact their speech development later in life. Ties can vary in severity, and the more severe tongue ties can lead to speech impairment because the tongue isn't free to move around the mouth to make the appropriate sounds for language development. So even if baby is successfully breastfeeding, consult with your health care provider if you are concerned about baby having a tongue or lip tie.

Coping With Common Challenges

Thrush

Thrush is a yeast infection that can manifest on the nipple. The bacteria that causes yeast infections naturally occurs in your body. When the other natural bacteria in your body are off-balance, the milk often left on your nipple following a breastfeeding session, combined with the moist, warm, and dark environment inside your shirt, contribute to the perfect environment for a yeast infection. Additionally, if you have to take antibiotics (for mastitis, for example), this may increase your risk of thrush. Antibiotics kill bacteria, good and bad. So, a round of antibiotics may throw off your body's natural balance. If you have to take an antibiotic while breastfeeding, discuss with your doctor how to potentially avoid thrush.

Oftentimes, pain associated with thrush only occurs during a letdown. In addition to the physical pain while breastfeeding, you may also notice that your nipples are pinker than normal or even shiny.

Thrush can also be present in your baby's mouth. If you notice white or light yellow splotches in baby's mouth (that can't be wiped off) and they seem uncomfortable, they likely have thrush. After my second son had his tongue tie cut, we soon developed thrush. Initially, I noticed white in his mouth that did not disappear when he swallowed, and he was incredibly fussy and frustrated while feeding. I then became super sore in both nipples, which made feeding, especially the initial latch, unbearable.

As with my baby, thrush can be passed from baby to mom and vice versa. So if you suspect you or baby has thrush, call up your healthcare provider so you can get antifungal medication to clear it up. One way you can possibly prevent thrush is by wiping your nipple following each nursing session and ensuring it's dry before you cover it up if you're wearing a bra or clothes that aren't loose fitting.

Chapped Nipples

As you work to establish your breastfeeding relationship with your baby and your baby works to nail the best latch, it's not uncommon for your breasts to become chapped, which can sometimes result in cracked nipples. As baby is trying to latch in the early days, they may chew on your nipple instead of placing the whole areola in their mouth. It's important to keep an eye on baby while they're breastfeeding to encourage a good latch. If you notice them not getting a good latch and they seem to be chewing on your nipple more than stimulating the areola, insert your pinky finger into the corner of their mouth. You want to get it between their gums and twist your hand to break their latch. Once you take them off the breast, take the steps we discussed earlier to encourage the correct latch. As your baby develops the correct latch through practice and your correction, your nipples should heal in no time! You can use nipple creams to help them heal. Another tip I learned was to place a little bit of expressed milk on the nipple and let it air dry following a nursing session. Thankfully, if you do end up getting chapped nipples, they heal pretty quickly and can be resolved by ensuring baby has a proper latch.

Low Milk Supply

When I was breastfeeding, there were times I was worried about my milk supply. Most new moms will worry about this at one point or another. Oftentimes, when baby is experiencing a growth spurt, it is not uncommon for them to want to feed more frequently. This is referred to as cluster feeding. Moms might worry that baby is feeding more because they aren't producing enough milk. But usually baby is cluster feeding to signal your body to make more milk to accommodate their growth spurt.

However, if you feel as though this may not be the case because your baby constantly seems hungry, has a drop in the number of diapers, or doesn't seem as satisfied following a nursing session, your milk supply could be dropping. Another indication might be if you're having to pump primarily (or exclusively), you may notice a reduction in your output when you pump.

If that's the case, there are some steps you can take to encourage your body to make more milk. The first thing to check for is if you're eating enough healthy calories. Also check your water input. If you're not staying hydrated, this can affect your milk production.

If you're eating and drinking enough, you could pump to encourage milk production. Remember that breast milk production is based on supply and demand. So, if you're noticing you're not producing as much, pump to signal your body that it needs to make more breast milk. You can pump between nursing sessions to ensure your breasts are completely empty once baby has fed. This can alert your body that it needs to increase its milk production.

Stress can also affect milk production. If you're feeling particularly stressed, try to focus on some self-care to help yourself unwind. Maybe a few hours from baby can help if you're overwhelmed with motherhood. If that's not possible, or being apart from baby will only add to your stress, a warm bath can help you unwind and destress as well.

If you take these steps and you find your supply is still lower than what you think your baby needs, you may consider supplementing with formula. Your health and well-being, as well as baby's, are the most important things. So, if you feel that your baby isn't getting everything they need from breastfeeding, there is no shame or judgment in supplementing with formula. The goal for new parents is a happy and healthy baby; this may mean that their nutrition comes from something other than your breast milk. Whatever you need to do to ensure your baby's needs are met is the right thing for you!

Hormones and Intimacy

Throughout your pregnancy and into postpartum while you're breastfeeding, your hormones are likely all over the place. These unpredictable hormones can absolutely impact your mood. The hormones from breastfeeding also can have the effect of decreasing your libido. This is nature's way of saying, "Wait a minute, you're not ready to conceive again!" While this is a natural defense of your body, it can be frustrating for you and your partner.

In addition to the changes inside your body, you're probably getting used to the changes outside your body. Some women bounce back to their pre-pregnancy bodies shortly after giving birth and feel great about themselves. I did not fall into this category! I was very conscious about the changes my body went through and didn't feel sexy at all. In addition to not being comfortable in your skin, your partner may view your body differently. They may see it as "baby's property."

Your partner may be trying to be respectful of you since you just had a baby, but you may worry that they don't find you attractive anymore. Once baby is born, make sure to keep communication open with your partner. Discuss what you're feeling and how you can meet each other's needs while respecting your new normal. In addition to all these changes, your breasts may be more sensitive or tender. Do what is right for you and be honest with your partner about what you need and how you feel.

Other Common Challenges and Making the Right Choice

When your milk first comes in, your breasts will most likely become engorged with milk, and they may feel tender or sore. I will never forget when I had my first baby. One of the nurses told me I'd feel like I had two bowling balls on my chest when my milk came in. Of course, everyone is different, but that was definitely the case with my first child. It was very obvious to me when my milk came in.

Breastfeeding baby with engorged breasts can present a challenge because it may make it difficult for baby to properly latch to draw out milk. If you find that's the case when your milk comes in, it may help to hand express (or use a pump if you have access to one) milk to remove some of it from your breast. If you do pump to relieve the engorgement, pump just enough to release the pressure. The goal is to help relax the breast so baby can properly (and comfortably) latch, not encourage your body to produce even more milk than you might need.

When you first experience your letdown, it can feel a bit strange. If your breasts are particularly full, it can even be somewhat painful or uncomfortable. Fortunately, letdowns don't typically last very long, so any discomfort from it passes quickly.

One thing to also be aware of is that breastfed babies can develop colic and reflux, just like formula-fed babies. If you discover that your baby is experiencing discomfort that isn't easily comforted by your soothing or breastfeeding, you can try different breastfeeding positions that may help bring them some relief. The laid back breastfeeding position is one that might bring baby relief if they're experiencing discomfort in their tummies.

Breastfeeding is a skill that will be brand new to you and your baby. Even if you've had other children you've successfully breastfed, each child is different. You may find that what worked for one baby may not work for another. As you navigate the breastfeeding journey, keep this in mind and do what works to ensure a happy and healthy baby and mommy. Whatever you need to do is worth it and is not something you should be ashamed of or judged for!

CHAPTER 11:

Evolving Appetites

—◆—

As your baby grows and gets bigger, you may notice changes in their feeding patterns and appetites. This is completely natural and to be expected!

Adapting to Your Growing Baby

With time, they will become more efficient at removing milk, and their stomach will grow. This means they will likely have longer periods between nursing sessions. Generally, you can expect them to begin to associate day and night, and transition to more feedings during the day. Hopefully, this translates to fewer nighttime feeds! As baby grows and is able to stay satisfied for longer, you'll likely see an improvement in their (and your) sleep at night. However, that doesn't mean they will completely sleep through the night. They'll still require some feedings at night, just not at the frequency of when they were a newborn. This also doesn't take into consideration waking at night due to discomfort. So, while you can expect to see a decrease in night feedings, don't expect to sleep through the night just yet!

Transition to Combination Feeding

Some moms might find themselves needing to explore combination feeding. This is when a baby is fed from the breast and a bottle. It can mean a mom who exclusively uses breast milk but feeds from the breast as well as the bottle, or it can mean a mom who has to feed baby formula in addition to breast milk. There could be a multitude of reasons why a mom needs to combination feed. Some moms may need to introduce a bottle because they need to return to work and can't exclusively nurse from the breast. Other moms may struggle with their supply and need to supplement with formula to ensure their baby is getting the nutrients they need, or they don't have the time to express but really want their baby to have a bottle at certain times of the day. Whatever ensures your baby is happy and healthy is what matters!

Doctors and lactation specialists recommend waiting to introduce a bottle until breastfeeding is established, if possible. This allows your baby to improve their latch and helps to establish your supply. Pumping breast milk can alert your body to make more milk, but a baby is generally going to be more effective at removing milk from the breast than a pump (whether mechanical or manual). If you can, establish the breastfeeding relationship within the first six to eight weeks, and then you can introduce combination feeding.

If you begin combination feeding with breast milk and formula, baby may gradually get more formula over time until eventually they stop breastfeeding. If that's what you need to do to feed your baby, you should not feel guilty or judged for it. Feeding your baby is a personal experience and decision, and only you know what's best for your breastfeeding dyad.

Navigating Nosy and Distractable Babies

As your baby grows, they become more alert and aware of their surroundings. All these new sights and sounds are so interesting to them! As they get bigger, they want to catalog and interact with these new sensations. This is great for their development but can be frustrating while they're breastfeeding because it's not uncommon for them to be curious and easily distracted while at the breast.

Earlier, we mentioned using scarves, shawls, or covers for discreet breastfeeding in public. But these can also serve the purpose of closing baby off from the world around them, thus minimizing distractions and encouraging them to focus on the task at hand: eating!

My babies were not fans of being covered while nursing. Instead of minimizing distractions, a cover served to distract them more because they became frustrated with having something over their head. If your baby is similar, consider trying to find a quiet space to breastfeed so they can complete their nursing session without additional distractions. If you're at someone's house, you can see if they have a spare room you can use, or if you're in public, some places have family rooms where you can sit and nurse baby in peace.

Another option is to bottle- or cup-feed baby expressed milk while you're on the go if you know your baby gets easily distracted. This option does require some planning and forethought, so it may not be as feasible.

If none of those options are available and it seems as though baby isn't going to make it through the full feeding session, don't get frustrated! One ineffective nursing session won't spell disaster for them. I know there have been times I've been so entrenched in something that I accidentally skipped lunch. Sure, I was hungry once I realized it, but I just ate as soon as I realized I missed my meal. The same thing goes for your baby. There may be times when you need to be more flexible. Minor disruptions in their feeding routine are completely normal, and they'll likely make up for it with more efficient feeds later on.

CHAPTER 12:

Feeding the Older Baby

—◆—

The only thing guaranteed in parenthood is that nothing will stay the same. Once you establish a successful breastfeeding relationship with your baby, you may run into some of the hurdles we previously discussed or some other natural developments that aren't hurdles but present a change in the routine you may have previously established with baby.

Transitioning to Solid Foods

Transitioning to solid food can be an exciting milestone for a family. It's bittersweet that your baby is growing up and gaining a sliver of independence. The American Academy of Pediatrics recommends that babies not receive solid food before six months (*Infant Food and Feeding*, 2021). Another good recommendation is to wait to introduce solid foods until baby is able to sit up unassisted and can control their neck and head.

Once your baby displays the signs indicating they're ready to try solid foods, a slow introduction is best. There is a saying that "food before one is just for fun." Once you start introducing other food to your baby, your breast milk still provides all the nutrients your baby needs. Just because baby is experimenting with solids, your breast milk's nutritional value doesn't decline. It helps to view solids as an exploratory phase. They won't be eating entire meals of solids once they hit six months. Allow them to play with their food as they discover new textures and flavors!

Mashed or soft foods are recommended as baby's first food because they're easy for them to consume. You can even mix things like oatmeal with expressed breast milk so baby has a familiar taste and texture with the new food. As your baby is exploring the different things you offer them, don't be alarmed if they cough or gag when eating. Around six months is when a baby's gag reflex isn't as sensitive. Prior to six months, it's a defense mechanism that can keep things out of their mouth that shouldn't be in there. Avoid giving baby small chunks of food that cannot be easily dissolved or gummed.

As you introduce food to your baby, try to only introduce one thing at a time. If baby has a reaction to something they ate, it's easier to determine what caused it if you're only introducing one new food at a time. If you kept a food journal when you began breastfeeding, it may be a good idea to keep one for baby when you start introducing them to solid food. It also helps if you wait a few days before introducing another new food item to ensure they don't have a delayed reaction to something they ate.

You may have noticed when you were breastfeeding that baby had an adverse reaction when you ate a certain food. For example, when I ate curry, I noticed my baby had a tummy ache. That doesn't necessarily mean they won't be able to handle the food they demonstrated a reaction to. You might just want to pay close attention when you do introduce those food items you know they had issues with through your breast milk.

Efficient Feeding and Comfort Nursing

Once baby establishes a successful latch, they become quite efficient at removing milk from the breast. It's not uncommon for older babies to be able to nurse for five minutes and be fully satisfied. They have the latch and suckling motion down, and their tummies have grown to accommodate a larger feeding.

One thing you may have had to do when baby was a newborn was to wake them to nurse. Now, as baby gets older, you may have to interrupt their playtime to nurse. They're becoming enamored with the world around them, so stopping to eat may not be high on their list of priorities.

As baby gets older, breastfeeding may bring them comfort in addition to nutrition. If baby is upset or gets hurt, breastfeeding them can have an amazing calming effect. The suckling motion combined with the warmth of your body and the sound of your voice can give baby the reassurance they need. Baby might also want to breastfeed more frequently if they don't feel well. Not only is your breast milk packed with nutrients to help them while they're sick, but breastfeeding can provide them comfort in the same way as mentioned above.

Some people might discourage you from breastfeeding baby for comfort, but that's their opinion. If you want to nurse your baby when they're upset or unwell, that's your prerogative. I breastfed my babies for both nutrition and comfort and they have grown up to be independent children who know I'm their safe home base. Their relationship with you is the first relationship a baby is exposed to. You get to determine how you want that relationship to look. Don't let strangers, friends, or family make you feel guilty or shame you for choosing to comfort your baby through breastfeeding.

Challenges of Reduced Milk Production

As mentioned before, breast milk is produced based on supply and demand. So, as baby feeds less, your body makes less milk. This is why it's important to continue to breastfeed them while you introduce solids. When I was introducing solids to my babies, our pediatrician recommended breastfeeding baby first and then giving them food. This ensured that baby was getting their fill nutritionally from my breast milk and the food was a bonus that helped them (and me) discover what they did and didn't like.

When baby was a newborn, it was probably easier to determine which breast to feed them on. Chances are, whichever breast they last nursed from would seem less "full." But as baby gets older, your supply evens out, and baby is feeding less frequently, so it may not be as easy to tell. When my babies got older, I noticed my breasts weren't as firm; they were softer because they weren't filling as much. If you want to continue switching sides but aren't sure how to keep track, some women will use a clothespin or something similar. Whichever side baby fed from last, they place the clothespin on that bra strap. That way, when baby's ready to nurse again, you know which side they last ate on. There are even breastfeeding apps, and keeping a written log can also be helpful. It can be more difficult to remember the older they get because they're probably going longer between nursing sessions, so it's not as fresh in your mind.

Teething

Once your baby starts teething, breastfeeding might be a little tricky. When they begin teething, their poor little gums are sore, and having suffered with just wisdom teeth as an adult, I can only imagine the discomfort they're in! Applying pressure to the gums can help to alleviate some of their discomfort, and some babies may apply pressure by biting or chewing on your nipple. Ouch! The only thing I really found that deterred that behavior was unlatching them and taking the nipple away when they did that. The goal was to teach them that if they bit the nipple that fed them, it would be taken away. I would offer the breast again after a few minutes, and if they bit me again, I'd take it away again. It didn't take them long to figure it out; babies are usually quick learners!

An easy way to provide baby some relief is to freeze some of your breast milk in a popsicle mold or something similar. When the milk is frozen, you can give it to baby to gnaw on. The cold helps alleviate their pain and the frozen milk allows them to put pressure on their gums. Plus, they get a little snack out of it too!

As your baby gets older, you'll discover that their needs change, which in turn may mean your breastfeeding relationship changes. Part of breastfeeding is about going with the flow and being flexible. Some milestones can be expected and prepared for, whereas others may take you by surprise. Whatever happens, stay in tune with your baby so you can meet them where they're at.

CHAPTER 13:

Toddlers and Weaning

—◆—

The Right Time to Stop

If you've breastfed your baby beyond the six-month mark and you've introduced other foods into their diet, you may begin to wonder when you should stop breastfeeding. As with all other decisions regarding breastfeeding, the decision of when to stop breastfeeding your child is a personal one.

Exclusively breastfeeding your baby for six months is encouraged as the best source of nutrition. Beyond six months, it's still recommended to continue breastfeeding so baby continues to receive the nutrients in the breast milk as they adapt to eating more solid foods. Beyond one year, breast milk does not lose any nutritional value. If your child is still removing milk from the breast regularly, your body will continue to produce milk to replace it.

As your child gets older, examine the breastfeeding relationship and determine when it would be best for you and your child to cease breastfeeding. Just like no one should make you feel bad for your choice to breastfeed, no one should make you feel bad for your decision to continue to breastfeed (or not!).

When you decide to bring breastfeeding to an end, you and your child may have feelings about it, and that's okay! You might be surprised that you're sad to end that physical connection your child has relied on for their life so far. Whether you celebrate the end of this milestone or mourn it, allow yourself to feel whatever emotions come along with it. And allow your child to experience it as well. It's a chapter of your lives that is coming to an end, so it's understandable that there will be some emotions surrounding it one way or another.

Transitioning to Toddlerhood

As your baby gets older, the breastfeeding relationship will undoubtedly change. Your child will likely begin to rely on solid food for their primary source of nutrition and won't need breast milk as frequently. This is the natural process of weaning.

Some toddlers may rely on breastfeeding in the mornings and evenings and possibly for nap time as well. If you're looking to cut those feedings out, consider replacing the breastfeeding session with something else. For example, if they wake up wanting to breastfeed, offer them a cup of cow's or alternative milk instead of breast milk. If you have extra breast milk stored, you could also offer them breast milk in a cup if your main focus is to wean them from nursing from the breast. Once you've depleted your supply, you'll need to transition them over to cows' or alternative milk.

If your child is used to nursing at bedtime, consider offering extra stories and snuggles without breastfeeding. As mentioned above, weaning is a great opportunity to teach your child about boundaries and respecting others' bodies.

Be gentle with yourself and your child if you're opting to wean them from the breast. They've become accustomed to having access to breast milk most parts of the day. So, it may be frustrating at first as you learn to set boundaries, but with time and persistence, you and your baby will be able to move past the breastfeeding relationship.

A tactic that I've used during the day to cut down on breastfeeding is distraction. Sometimes, my child would want to nurse, and instead of engaging, I would offer a different activity they could do, such as drawing, coloring, or playing with toys. This helped move their mind to other activities they could engage in.

If you become pregnant while you're breastfeeding, your breastfeeding child may naturally stop breastfeeding on their own without any need from you to intervene. Oftentimes, when a woman becomes pregnant while breastfeeding, they will see a drop in their milk supply. This may lead to your child breastfeeding less simply because there isn't much there or they have to work harder to get milk. Additionally, sometimes the flavor of the breast milk will change when you become pregnant, so this could be another reason a child may not want to continue breastfeeding.

Challenges of Toddler Weaning

One of the challenges that you might encounter with weaning your toddler is how vocal they might be. My daughter would often try to pull my sweater up while we were in public and shout "boobies" when she wanted to nurse. This can cause some anxiety for you if they're older and you're not completely comfortable with nursing them beyond what is seen as "normal" breastfeeding age in society!

Toddlers also aren't great at being told no. If you're breastfeeding a toddler and they ask in public but you say no, chances are you now get to try to manage a meltdown. But the good news is that most mothers have had to deal with toddler meltdowns in public, whether it's breastfeeding related or not! So just know that you're not alone and that every mother who goes into public with their child will likely experience this. As I mentioned earlier, distraction can be a really effective tactic for redirecting a toddler.

Many women find themselves contemplating weaning or stopping breastfeeding due to societal pressures. But if your baby is older than a year old and you find that continuing breastfeeding suits you, there is no reason to stop.

With older children, sometimes breastfeeding is more of a comfort. It can be a way for your child to ground themselves when situations become overwhelming.

So far, I've breastfed my third child, my daughter, for the longest. At two and a half, she was still nursing at bedtime and occasionally first thing in the morning. I was pregnant and had been planning to stop her before her little brother arrived. However, he arrived unexpectedly eight weeks early, and I remained in the hospital. Suddenly, I wasn't there, so the poor thing went cold turkey without nursing. When I finally came home, she didn't ask for it, which was such a relief as I needed the milk for the baby.

Gradual Weaning for Minimal Discomfort

As you begin your weaning journey, you may experience some discomfort depending on when you opt to wean your child. If your child is still relatively young (under a year old) and milk dependent, you may discover some discomfort as you wean. The best course for weaning at this stage is to do so gradually. You can begin by cutting out one nursing session at a time and giving your body (and baby) some time to adjust. For example, cut out one nursing session and wait a day or two before cutting out the next one. As your baby removes less milk from the breast, your body will receive the signal to produce less milk. This will allow for a more gradual process for you and baby. If you try to stop suddenly while your baby is still milk dependent, it will be jarring to them as well as your body. You're more likely to experience engorgement in the breasts if you stop suddenly.

If you're breastfeeding your child beyond a year old and they're less milk dependent, you might discover that your breasts don't feel as full as often as they did in the early days of breastfeeding. Some mothers worry that this means their bodies aren't making as much milk to match their nursing child's needs. But that only means your body has discovered how much your baby needs and doesn't produce more than necessary. If you opt to gradually wean at this stage as well, your body will gradually reduce how much milk it makes without the stimulation from your baby removing milk from the breast.

However you choose to begin the weaning process, remember to focus on what is best for you and your baby. Weaning is a personal decision that only you can make. Once you've weaned your child, you may still be able to express small amounts of milk for a few months once your baby has stopped nursing. This is perfectly normal and will eventually cease altogether.

CHAPTER 14:

Looking After Momma

—◆—

Prioritizing "Me Time"

If this is your first baby, you may not be familiar with the toll motherhood can take on you. If this is not your first baby, you may be aware that since becoming a mother, you've lost touch with yourself and seemingly your identity as an individual. Motherhood is a full-time job, and when you add breastfeeding to it, it can become a labor-intensive one as well.

The transition to motherhood can be fast, furious, and overwhelming. You may not realize that you feel like you're losing your sense of self until you're burned out and run down. Being a primary caregiver requires a lot of time, energy, attention, and dedication. This can take away from the time you devote to yourself, and you may not realize the impact it has on you because it's not something you've had to think about before.

When you breastfeed, it can be difficult to enlist the help of a partner, especially if your baby is nursing straight from the breast and you're not pumping. The best advice I can offer is, in the early stages, to ask your partner for help, if possible, and make time for yourself.

In current society, "self-care" is often seen as extravagant acts of indulgence. That's not what I'm talking about, though. I'm referring to the most basic of ways you can take care of yourself. Oftentimes, when we're in the primary caregiver role, we ensure everyone's needs are met before ours. But if you've ever been on a plane, you know the flight attendants will instruct you to affix your oxygen mask before putting it on small children. The same principle applies to taking care of yourself. You need to ensure your physical, emotional, and basic needs are being met before you can tend to those around you. So, make sure you're eating healthy, staying hydrated, and getting enough sunshine. It may sound silly but when you tend to your needs, it makes it easier to focus on what those around you need.

Part of self-care is taking additional time for yourself outside of your role as a mother or caregiver. With breastfeeding, you spend a lot of time physically attached to your baby (especially in the early days). One thing I learned the hard way was that moms can absolutely become "touched out." Because of your baby's physical need to be with you all the time, you may get to a point where you don't want to be touched at all. This is your signal to take some time away without anyone or anything needing your attention. Ideally, you would carve out time so you don't get to that point.

It could be something as simple as turning over nonfeeding-related duties to your partner and going on a walk or reading alone for a given amount of time. Only you know what your body needs. Unfortunately, there isn't a scientific equation that outlines how much "me time" you might need to balance with your role as a mom or caregiver. Listen to your body and learn what you need in order to continue to provide the care your family needs from you.

Communication with your partner in this regard is also important. Let them know you need time to yourself to recoup and recover from the demands placed on you. Oftentimes, partners who are not in the primary caregiver role naturally get time to rest and recover, so they may not realize that time needs to be carved out for you to be able to do the same.

You're not selfish for needing "me time." You're a human with basic needs, and sometimes, we have to advocate for those needs to be met if we're feeling burned out or touched out. There is nothing wrong with that! One of the dichotomies of motherhood is that you can feel resentful for not having time to yourself, but then, if you do get time away, you feel guilt for enjoying it. Another thing to remember is to allow yourself to feel those feelings! Motherhood can be complicated, but as you find your way, embrace those feelings and use them to inform yourself of where you can support yourself by reaching out to others.

And something to keep in mind is that "me time" is not simply time spent away from your breastfeeding baby. So, while laundry, dishes, or grocery shopping are things done without your baby, you're still fulfilling your role as caregiver in those tasks. As you explore carving out "me time," consider looking at things you enjoy doing that give you a rush of dopamine that have nothing to do with your role as a mother or caregiver.

Rediscovering Hobbies

As a new mom, you may hear the words "hobbies" and laugh. I know I did. In the early days of breastfeeding, it may seem laughable that you have any extra time to focus on anything other than your baby. But as you fall into a routine, consider reclaiming your "me time" with some things you enjoyed before you had your baby. Again, it doesn't have to be something extravagant or require tons of money or time. What are some things you enjoyed before that can be easily incorporated into your daily life once again? I enjoy reading, and that's relatively easy to do while baby is sleeping or something I can sneak away and do to get a chapter read.

Before you became a mom, you had likes, dislikes, wants, and needs that all culminated into your identity. One common complaint with moms is that once they have children, they lose their sense of self and their identity. Look back at what made you who you are before you had children. Sure, some of that might change slightly because you have a family to care for. Maybe you used to enjoy overnight hiking trips, and that's something that would require extensive planning. But what are some things you enjoyed before having your child(ren) that you can still do while requiring relatively little planning or orchestrating?

As you rediscover the things you once enjoyed, you can even potentially involve your family if you so desire. Sharing the things we enjoy with those we love can help them see you as an individual as well as add to the quality time you spend together. With the example of hiking above, taking an overnight hiking trip with little ones may not be feasible (or more work than it's worth!), but a day hiking trip may be something you can more easily enjoy with your family.

Rediscovering your hobbies is about revisiting that which brought you joy before you became a mother. It's not meant to be isolating, though. Some mothers may prefer to isolate themselves with their hobbies just to give them a break from their duties and responsibilities, which is completely understandable and something I have done! But as you are able to balance your "me time" with your role as caregiver, you can begin to explore ways to include your family in your hobbies if that's something you'd like to do.

Carving out time for yourself and engaging in hobbies you once enjoyed are just a couple of ways you can keep your cup full so you can continue to fill the cups of those around you.

Exercising and Nurturing Relationships

Exercise is something that can help you carve out that "me time" and refocus on your physical needs. Some moms might have enjoyed exercising before motherhood and may have stopped for fear of causing their baby harm. But once you've had your baby, your doctor will often give you the green light to resume physical activity six weeks following giving birth. If you had a C-section, this may be eight weeks as you allow your incision to heal.

There is no reason you can't exercise while exclusively breastfeeding your baby. One of the main things to remember if you begin exercising is to stay hydrated. Hydration is important to breastfeeding, so if you're working out, you want to ensure you're consuming enough water for what you may be expending.

Whether you were running half marathons before you gave birth or a nice walk around the block was your idea of a workout, you want to take it easy. Start slow and listen to your body. If your body was used to rigorous workouts before you became pregnant, you've basically been out of commission for almost a year, so you'll need to ease back into your workout routine.

As you begin a routine, listen to the cues your body gives you. If you're tired, don't push yourself beyond what you're able to do. Consider starting with a walk around the block just to gauge how your body feels as you become in tune with it. If the walk around the block was tough, shorten the distance next time you go out. Or if it was a breeze, add distance in small increments. Remember, you're trying to build your physical body, so not listening to it will only likely set you back as you get back on your feet.

As you explore what kind of physical activities you like and enjoy, consider acquiring supportive sports bras if you don't already have any. You want to be sure the sports bra fits well without fitting too tightly. As with regular bras, additional pressure on the breast tissue can potentially lead to clogged milk ducts. If you had sports bras before you became pregnant, I would recommend getting some new ones that would be able to accommodate your changing breasts. You want a sports bra that isn't overly restricting and will allow you to move freely. You might also want to look into sports bras specifically designed for breastfeeding. These can provide the needed support while allowing ease for feeding when necessary.

In addition to finding time for yourself and meeting your physical needs, it's also important to carve out time to spend with your partner. Just like you had your own identity before you became a mother, your relationship with your partner had its own unique dynamic before you both became parents. Not fostering that connection and touching base with each other regularly can lead to a breakdown in the relationship. It's important to show each other that despite the changes in your life, you're still priorities to each other. As mentioned above, communication is incredibly important here. Your partner may feel bad about asking for your time because they see how you're stretching yourself for the family, but you both need to know that maintaining that connection with each other is incredibly important at this time. You need to be advocates and supporters of each other and your relationship. Remind yourselves what brought you together in the first place and allow for space in your lives to keep that relationship strong and alive.

CHAPTER 15:

My Personal Experience

—◆—

The advice in this book comes from my own experience as I navigated motherhood and breastfeeding with four babies. The women in my family are all prolific breastfeeders. So, it was never a question of "if" I would breastfeed. They made it look so easy and natural, so I never even considered any other options or alternatives. I did do a little bit of research, and with suggestions from family, I purchased some nursing bras and breast pads. Beyond that, I figured I didn't need to do any further research because I was genetically inclined to breastfeed, right?

Arthur—A Rocky Start

Not entirely right. My oldest child was born three weeks early. I had to be induced after my water broke, and once he was born, it became evident that breastfeeding didn't always "just happen." Because he was born three weeks early, the nurses surmised that he had not yet developed the sucking reflex, which, as you can imagine, is quite important in breastfeeding. I had no idea what I was doing, and apparently, neither did my poor baby.

The midwives in the hospital didn't let me give up on the chance to breastfeed my baby. They spent time encouraging me and, quite frankly, manhandling me (once you have a baby, any sense of modesty and dignity often flies out the window when you're in the hospital). They intervened to show me how to help him properly latch and how to keep him awake and eating when he was tired and just wanted to sleep. They also reminded me that because of his size, it was important that I wake him up to nurse him because he was such a sleepy baby he likely wouldn't wake up on his own to eat. Without their help and support, I'm not sure I would have been able to continue my breastfeeding journey with Arthur. After spending a couple of days at the birthing center, I was confident we had the hang of this breastfeeding thing.

Despite our rocky start, Arthur became a proficient feeder. He fed regularly throughout the day, and much to my surprise, he even slept through the night at six weeks! Everything seemed to go well and without incident. Once we established our breastfeeding relationship, Arthur seemed to be the perfect complement to our breastfeeding dyad. He even adapted to nursing in public well; he developed his own way of watching the world while staying attached to the breast.

I was fortunate not to suffer from mastitis or any of the other issues common with breastfeeding. I did, however, experience chapped nipples since my nipples weren't used to being used so extensively! Nipple creams were a lifesaver in those early days, and once my nipples adjusted, I haven't had any issues nursing any of my babies since.

After we celebrated six weeks of Arthur being outside the womb, I began to express breast milk once Arthur finished with his morning feeding. I started out using a manual pump. But after doing this for many days in a row, my hands began to ache. Thankfully, I had a friend who had an electric pump they no longer needed, so they let me use it.

With my morning pumping session and the electric pump, I was able to pump seven ounces each day from just one session. I often worried about how much milk Arthur was receiving while he nursed, so I would give him the seven-ounce bottle at bedtime that I'd pumped that morning to make myself feel better, knowing he was getting a sufficient feed. In hindsight, I realize his weight gain and regular growth were all indicators that he was receiving enough milk from me without having to give him a bottle in the evening. But being a new mom, I felt better about knowing how much he was getting at night.

A perk of introducing a bottle earlier on was that it was a relief to know he'd easily take a bottle if needed (if I had to leave him with someone besides myself for any reason), and it also made weaning easier. Arthur also took a pacifier, which was a relief because I knew he wasn't using nursing as a comfort; it was strictly to get the nutrients he needed.

By the time Arthur was eight months old, he was eating solid foods three times a day and receiving milk four times a day. When he reached nine months, I became pregnant with my next child. The beginning of the pregnancy had me feeling unwell, so having Arthur take a bottle made my life so much easier at this stage. Around this time, we stopped breastfeeding, and while it was emotional, I felt as though we had a very successful journey and it was the right time for us to stop. I was especially proud of how far we'd come despite our rocky start. It was also around this time that Arthur started his first sessions at nursery as I prepared to go back to work.

Charles—Navigating Tongue Tie, Thrush, and Mastitis

Charles was born one week early, and the difference between his birth and establishing the breastfeeding relationship was night and day from that with Arthur! My delivery with Charles went quickly and without any complications. Once he was born, I was able to latch him right away, and he seemed to get the hang of breastfeeding without any issues. But when he was born, it was discovered that he had a tongue tie, as mentioned in a previous chapter. This is when the skin underneath the tongue is more attached, preventing the tongue from moving freely while breastfeeding. When it was discovered, it was recommended I have the tongue tie cut (which is a common remedy for this issue). We made an appointment to have this taken care of when he was three weeks old. In the meantime, we settled into a routine. Charles fed well, and we began to have longer gaps between feedings at night and during the day.

When it came time for his appointment, we attended as planned. The doctors explained to me that they would simply cut the piece of skin that was restricting his tongue from moving freely. They assured me that it would be like an injection; he would feel a scratch, and then it would be over. You can imagine I had my doubts!

It was difficult to watch them as they tried to hold him down and open his mouth to be able to perform the "simple" procedure. And, of course, my poor three-week-old wasn't a willing participant, making it all that more difficult by fighting them each step of the way. I would never have imagined a doctor and nurse would struggle to restrain a three-week-old for a "simple" procedure!

As promised, the doctor made the cut very quickly, and Charles stopped crying shortly after. I was a whole other story. I think it was more traumatizing for me than for him. It just goes to show how resilient babies truly are. I wasted no time whisking him away to nurse him and offer him comfort in the best way I knew how.

While we had fallen into a comfortable routine prior to the procedure, I knew he would likely need some time to adjust to nursing without the previous restriction. It didn't take him long at all to get used to having a more mobile tongue.

Unfortunately, not long after this, Charles and I developed thrush. I was familiar with uncomfortable nipples from my time breastfeeding his brother, Arthur, but this was something else entirely. This wasn't just discomfort; this was awful pain. My nipples were in pain and it was agonizing trying to feed him. I began to further realize something wasn't right when Charles began to express discomfort while breastfeeding and an inability to settle. At one point, he was crying, and I noticed a small white blob inside his mouth. At first, I thought it was spit up. But upon further inspection, I couldn't wipe it away, and no matter how much I wiped it, it didn't budge.

The midwife came for a visit, and I asked her about it. She told me it was fine and most likely nothing to worry about. While I respect medical professionals, my mom instinct was telling me it was something to be worried about, so I went with my gut and spoke to a doctor. The doctor prescribed a vial of medicine. I was to drop the medicine into Charles's mouth, but I was not prescribed anything. At this point, I was an emotional mess. I took it upon myself to improvise. Once I placed the correct number of drops in Charles's mouth, I wiped the excess medicine from the side of the dropper around my nipples. I figured if it was good enough to heal the inside of Charles's mouth, it ought to be good enough to hopefully provide me some relief. Thankfully, this helped both of us, and my nipples and Charles's mouth healed.

Not long after this, I had my first experience with mastitis. I experienced flu-like symptoms and achy breasts with a localized sore red area, but I didn't make the connection that it could be mastitis. I just thought I was coming down with something.

As soon as I realized it was mastitis, I made sure to wear the loosest tops and most comfortable nursing bras. I also noticed that one particular spot on my breast was tender and red and realized this was likely the culprit. On one particular day that was really awful, a friend came over and picked up Arthur to take him to a playdate. With Arthur in the care of someone else, I got Charles settled down. I then took some pain relievers and drew a warm bath.

Over the next couple of days, I continued to nurse Charles as usual, and having him nurse on the affected breast helped to provide some relief. Within a few days, I started to feel better, and the mastitis cleared up.

Charles and I continued our breastfeeding journey, and it became clear from very early on that he was a nosy baby. Even just nursing him at home, he would get easily distracted by his brother, Arthur, playing in the same room. I figured that because of this, feeding him in public would be practically impossible.

Despite knowing this, it didn't stop me from trying. I had one particularly embarrassing moment while at a café. The tables were situated quite close together, and Charles had just settled in to start feeding. A gentleman next to us in a smart blazer waved and said a jolly "Hello!" to an approaching friend. Charles whipped his head away from my breast to investigate what was happening. Well, as luck would have it, my letdown had just kicked in and was flowing. A better description might be that my letdown was *spraying*. All over the arm of this poor gentleman's smart blazer. I frantically grabbed at the muslin blanket that was tucked under Charles. Given his nosy nature, I should have been better prepared and had the muslin draped over him before we got settled in. But, as they say, hindsight is twenty-twenty, and that is a lesson I learned the hard way.

As with many new mothers, I was very diligent when it came to taking Arthur to the local baby weighing clinic. I was a regular there and would strip him down, get him weighed, and talk to a healthcare worker about any concerns that may have cropped up. I made sure to religiously plot his growth and felt a surge of pride when I was told he was progressing along his lines as expected. Well, with Charles, I took him quite regularly soon after he was born, but I didn't take him as often as I took Arthur. Charles also progressed nicely along the developmental chart.

Quite some time passed between visits at the clinic, and I decided I ought to take him for a checkup. Charles was weighed by one of the healthcare workers, and to my surprise, not only had he fallen off his developmental progression, but he'd fallen to a much lower level. The healthcare worker directed me to sit with her at her desk, and once I was settled in, she asked me, "What has been going on?"

I felt like I was a child being called into the principal's office. I was devastated. She informed me that I needed to wake him every two hours—day and night—to feed him, despite the fact that he had begun sleeping for six-hour stretches at night. She instructed me to supplement his breast milk with formula as my milk must not be enough for him. Furthermore, she told me that if I insisted on continuing to breastfeed him, I had to feed him for twenty minutes on each side! I felt awful and so guilty that I had not realized he wasn't putting on weight.

I did my due diligence and bought formula at the healthcare worker's insistence. Try as I might, Charles completely refused the bottle and would only nurse from the breast. He also refused to eat for twenty minutes. If you've ever breastfed a baby, you know how impossible it is to force a baby to actively nurse if they're no longer hungry. Both of my babies only ever ate from one breast during a feeding. No matter how hard I tried, Charles wasn't interested in nursing from both breasts, let alone for twenty minutes.

I did, however, wake him up every two hours to feed him. He ended up gaining weight quickly, and he was a content and inquisitive baby. Honestly, I never went back to that clinic. As a breastfeeding mom, being berated did not help my mental state.

I tried the tactic I used with Arthur when he was a baby. I would express milk daily and prepare him a bottle to try to get Charles used to taking breast milk from the bottle. But with two young children, I typically was too busy with the two little ones or too distracted to remember to pump every single day. Because of this, he didn't end up getting a bottle every day like Arthur. But I did start bringing a bottle with me when we would go out in public. I quickly learned that if we were in public, he would take the bottle if he was allowed to feed himself. So that was a relief!

After Charles turned six months old, I started to introduce follow-on milk into his daytime feedings, so I was able to forgo expressing. He would still breastfeed first thing in the morning, before he went to sleep, and throughout the day. But by introducing the follow-on milk, I wasn't stressing about making sure he had enough. I also followed the healthcare worker's orders and woke him up every two hours, even at night. Even once he gained sufficient weight, trying to get him to break the habit of waking every two hours at night was nearly impossible.

By nine months old, Charles was still waking up to feed multiple times throughout the night. He took a pacifier, but he would still use me as one at night. He wouldn't necessarily need to feed when he woke up, but he would only calm when I put him to my breast. I stayed with my grandma (one of the prolific breastfeeders) at one point, and I—emotionally—told her I didn't know what to do because I was just so darn tired from waking up throughout the night with Charles. She was the one to tell me that there was no way he needed to be waking up to nurse that often at night with how old he was. She encouraged me to give him the pacifier when he woke up and refuse him the breast. Of course, she made it sound so simple! That night, I decided to give it a go with her emotional support behind me. He woke up, and instead of offering him the breast, I told him no and snuggled him instead. Much to my surprise, he actually went back to sleep with little effort. That then marked the end of our breastfeeding journey.

Rebecca—Coping with Reflux and Ongoing Feeding

Rebecca was my third baby, and she was born five days early. I was induced because my water broke, and her delivery went by very rapidly once they hooked me up to the induction drip. Once she was born, she latched onto the breast with no problems and began feeding right away. However, her lungs contained quite a bit of mucus, which the doctors surmised was a result of my labor and her subsequent delivery progressing so quickly. They explained that typically, while a mother is pushing, the action works to help expel the mucus from the baby's lungs. But since I didn't spend a lot of time pushing, this didn't happen. The first few days following her birth, she was quite sick because of the mucus, and it gave her a stomach ache.

If I had any doubts about whether she was consuming my colostrum, those were expelled at a pediatric visit. The morning after she was born, a doctor came in for a visit, and she vomited all over herself, and it was all colostrum. The pediatrician saw this as a good thing because not only did it indicate that her body was working to get rid of the mucus, but it also showed how much colostrum she expressed from breastfeeding.

Once we got home, she continued to demonstrate proficiency with breastfeeding, but after a few weeks, she developed reflux. Thankfully, it appeared to only be a mild version, but she would get sick if we laid her down too quickly following breastfeeding. The most immediate solution was to keep her upright for as long as possible after nursing her. At night, I was often sitting up with her until I couldn't keep my eyes open anymore. During the day, I didn't mind it so much as it was the perfect excuse to cuddle her—as if anyone needs an excuse to cuddle a baby.

I was a bit worried about the amount of milk she would spit up, concerned that she wasn't keeping enough down. To assuage my fears, my partner got a glass of water one day and spilled the smallest amount. It looked like quite a bit when it was spilled, but when I saw how much was actually displaced from the glass, I realized it really wasn't that much at all. This demonstration helped me relax.

Rebecca never really got attached to any comfort objects. She never took a pacifier, and as a toddler, she really only used it to chew on. It seemed nursing was her only comfort. We didn't really see an issue with this until it became apparent that we couldn't leave her with someone else.

Something else that was different with Rebecca was that she was sensitive to some foods I ate while I was breastfeeding her. For example, if I had a garlic-y curry, the next day, she would appear to be uncomfortable, loudly whining and having explosive diapers. As soon as I realized my food choices impacted her, I was careful to avoid foods that would upset her.

From about seven weeks, Rebecca slept through the night, and I was pretty smug about that. I enjoyed some wonderful restful nights. That is until we all caught COVID-19 when she was about seven months old. She was incredibly sick and uncomfortable. The only thing that seemed to help her through the night was nursing and being held by either my partner or me. This went on for about a week, and unfortunately, once she was better, she still did not go back to sleeping through the night. I decided not to fight it, and I would lie down with her in my bed, nurse her, and let her stay there as we both fell asleep. I specifically remember the first time I gave in after a rocky time sleep-wise, and I felt so well rested after keeping her in bed with us. From then on, it became a habit for her to sleep in our bed. We eventually got to a place where she would start out sleeping in her bed and come into our bed whenever she woke up during the night. This didn't bother me or my partner and worked for us. We figured that as long as everyone was getting the sleep they needed, it didn't feel like much of a problem.

Rebecca was also pretty easy to nurse in public. She was a nosy baby like her brother, but she managed to focus on her task at hand and get through a nursing session with no problem. The ease with which I nursed her in public could also be attributed to the fact that she was my third breastfeeding baby, and I was more relaxed and less worried about accidentally flashing someone!

While I would nurse Rebecca, I would use the "milk catchers" to create a stash of milk in the freezer. I would then end up using this milk for her breakfasts once she started on solids. Rebecca never did take a bottle, which meant there was no flexibility in our breastfeeding relationship. This wasn't a problem because there weren't any instances in which I wasn't able to be with her during a feeding. If I had needed to be away from her for extended periods of time, I would have made more of an effort to ensure she took a bottle. But since it wasn't necessary, I chose not to pick that battle with her.

Rebecca continued to breastfeed until she was two years old. She would nurse before going to bed, if she woke in the night, and sometimes first thing in the morning. But by the end, she wasn't nursing during the day at all. But that all changed when my water abruptly broke at 31 weeks when I was pregnant with our fourth child. I was admitted to the hospital, and that was her first time away from me overnight. Since she never took a bottle, she had to quit nursing cold turkey as I was in the hospital. She seemed to handle it pretty well, only getting upset at bedtime when she wanted me and "boobies." I was somewhat surprised once I was discharged from the hospital that she never asked to nurse again. I think the transition was made a little easier because I was pumping every three hours for the new baby, and since she'd never seen me pump before, it was a little weird for her. We also talked about how I was collecting milk to give to her baby brother, who was in the hospital.

Philip—Overcoming a Scary Start

As I mentioned above, my water broke when I was 31 weeks pregnant with Philip. I had a particularly stressful pregnancy and was never able to really relax or enjoy it. Since I had never experienced preterm labor or delivering any of my babies prematurely, I was a terrified, panicky mess. Once I was admitted to the hospital, they administered antibiotics to stave off infection, as well as steroids to help the baby's lungs mature. I was then playing the waiting game to see if I went into labor naturally or if I would be able to be discharged and put on bed rest. The ultimate goal was to keep me pregnant for as long as possible, as even another week in utero would immensely benefit the baby's development.

Unfortunately, as this was a stressful pregnancy, the birth didn't go any easier. I ended up having an infection (Strep B) and went into labor. When they examined me, it was determined that I was dilating, but his feet were presenting first, so I was taken for an emergency C-section.

Once he was born, we were both in poor health. I was treated for sepsis, and Philip was diagnosed with pneumonia. He was immediately taken to the neonatal intensive care unit (NICU), where they tended to him wonderfully and helped him through a rough couple of days in the beginning. Initially, he was given nutrients through fluid via a line directly into his umbilical cord. After a few days, he received my milk for the first time, but it was delivered with a syringe through a nasogastric (NG) tube directly to his stomach.

As soon as he was born, the doctors encouraged me to pump since I wouldn't be able to feed him directly from the breast. Pumping helped my milk come in, signaling to my body that it needed to produce milk. The doctors told me the best medicine for Philip would be my breast milk, or magic milk, as they took to calling it.

I originally had my heart set on a vaginal delivery, preferably at home. So, the events that unfolded and left me sick and in the hospital led me to feel like my body had failed my baby. Despite knowing that C-sections are regularly performed and are just another way to bring a baby into this world, I was terrified of the surgery. But reason was nowhere to be found when I was a traumatized, hormonal mother. To add to that, I was bound to my room, only able to get around with assistance, and on the same floor as other new mothers with their babies, hearing the newborns cry while mine wasn't with me. In hindsight, while I was feeling pretty horribly sitting in my room, I had round-the-clock access to the NICU, and I was in there as often as I could be. They only asked me to leave when I was falling asleep next to him.

I spent the first few days after his birth in my head, berating myself and taking the blame for our situation. To top it off, my milk was nonexistent. This frustrated me because I was still breastfeeding his sister, Rebecca, up until my water broke at 31 weeks. This only added to my stress and confusion. One of the wonderful nurses attending to my son gave me a stern talking to. She reminded me about the importance of being kind to myself during this trying time, as well as reminding me that what happened was not my fault. This pep talk led to me giving myself some grace and a little extra self-love. And lo and behold, my milk came in the next day. By the time we left the NICU, I had even filled their freezer with a surplus of breast milk.

While he was in the NICU, they gradually increased his tube feeds, and once he was safely off all breathing apparatuses and the lines came out of his umbilical cord, I was able to try and breastfeed him. Thankfully, he picked it up really quickly, and once we established a solid breastfeeding foundation, we were able to return home. Because he was so little, I had to exert a little more energy to keep him engaged while breastfeeding. It didn't take much to tire him out and fall asleep, so I was using lots of chin and feet tickles and diaper changes to keep him awake and alert for his feedings.

Unfortunately for us, a week after having been discharged from the hospital, Philip picked up RSV. I took him to the hospital because he was not eating and struggling to eat. He needed oxygen for a couple of days, and he was once again fitted for an NG tube. But his feedings were stopped, and they opted to give him fluids instead to help maximize his lung capacity (full stomachs can reduce the lung capacity).

His health continued to deteriorate, so he was ventilated and transferred to a specialist hospital. He was on the ventilator for about six days before he was taken off it. Thankfully, he only needed oxygen for a few hours following being taken off the ventilator. They resumed his feedings, but they needed to measure how much he was taking in, which led to him having his first bottle of my expressed breast milk.

The doctors warned me that he might likely lose the reflex and ability to breastfeed. However, after receiving measured bottles for a few days, we were able to try him feeding from the breast. It quickly became apparent that he was unable to latch properly onto my breast, and when he did suck, it wasn't quite the same (indicating he wasn't extracting milk with the same efficiency he was able to previously).

I refused to give up, though. When it came time to feed him, I first offered him the breast so he could try to reacclimate himself to breastfeeding. It ended up with me giving him a bottle of expressed milk when he wasn't able to latch and express milk on his own. Once he finished feeding, I would pump milk for his next feeding. This went on for six weeks. Some days were better than others with his attempts at breastfeeding. Due to the amount I was pumping, I ended up with mastitis. The time I was devoting to pumping and feeding Philip was a real struggle as I had three other children who needed me as well, not to mention the commitments that come along with having two small children.

Toward the end of the six weeks, something seemed to just click with Philip, and he once again was nursing from the breast efficiently. It got to the point where he would refuse the top-up bottle I would offer him after nursing from the breast. I contacted my local Infant Feeding Team, and after consulting with them, I stopped offering the top-up bottle. For my peace of mind, I purchased some infant weighing scales to keep a close eye on his weight and ensure he was getting enough with my breast milk. I also kept an eye on any signs he might still be hungry once he was done nursing, as well as on his diapers, using them as an indicator that he had as much output as was to be expected. His weight continued to progress, and he is now breastfeeding well.

Final Thoughts and Advice

Throughout my breastfeeding journeys with my children, I learned that no two babies are the same. We had some rough patches, but we also had things worth celebrating. One thing that became evident was that it's important to do what works for you and your family. If you encounter an issue while breastfeeding, explore ways to fix it and do what you need to. Not everyone will agree with how you go about your breastfeeding journey, but it's yours, not theirs. I know that some might chastise me for having my daughter sleep in the bed with us, but it was what worked for us at the time. As I mentioned, when it comes to breastfeeding and children, we often have to pick and choose which battles we will engage in. I knew that my daughter wouldn't be in our bed forever and it wasn't detrimental to our lives for her to sleep with us if that was what she needed.

No matter what you choose to do (or not to do), all that matters is that your baby is fed and healthy. Whether you choose to feed formula, breast milk, or a combination of the two, only you know what's truly best for your baby and your family. Just like every baby is different, every breastfeeding journey will be different. Just because another mom has a baby who has a similar temperament to one of my children, that doesn't mean they're going to have a similar journey to us. Motherhood is about supporting each other through the hard times and celebrating the good times. When a mother and her baby have a successful breastfeeding relationship, it can be magical. But that isn't always the case, and mothers should never feel guilty for the hard times.

CHAPTER 16:

Moms' Circle of Strength

—◆—

While I came from a family of prolific breastfeeders, one of the things I found solace in during the rocky parts of my breastfeeding journey was support in different forms. Adequate and encouraging support can make all the difference in empowering a mother to continue breastfeeding despite obstacles.

Seeking Professional Help

Lactation consultants are truly the unsung heroes in a mother's breastfeeding journey. They are healthcare professionals who have been certified and trained in breastfeeding. They're often utilized to assist mothers when they have difficulty breastfeeding. Some hospitals and birthing centers will employ lactation consultants, so they're readily available to new mothers. Other lactation consultants have a private practice, so they're available even once you've left the hospital or birthing center. Because of their expertise, lactation consultants are familiar with common breastfeeding issues and can offer practical solutions for resolving these issues. Their goal is to ensure a positive experience for mothers and babies as they establish a breastfeeding relationship. Some of the ways lactation consultants can help include diagnosing and resolving latching issues and diagnosing and resolving pain while breastfeeding. While they're most commonly utilized in the first few weeks after a baby is born, they can also provide support once a mother has established a successful breastfeeding relationship with her baby.

Hospital and Midwifery Support

Midwives and nurses are also invaluable advocates in the labor, birth, and breastfeeding journey. If your hospital or birthing center has a midwife available, I would highly recommend utilizing their support. Midwives tend to be very hands on, encouraging laboring moms with various positions that help increase their comfort during labor. Then, once the baby is born, their focus is on ensuring baby is healthy and can assist with establishing that first feeding session immediately after the baby is born. They can help new moms experiment with different breastfeeding positions to ensure mom and baby are both comfortable, which will lead to a less stressed-out mom, encouraging her body to relax. Midwives are also adept at recognizing and addressing any issues that may crop up in those first twenty-four to forty-eight hours following the birth of the baby. Where lactation consultants specialize in breastfeeding, midwives are healthcare professionals with vast knowledge and insight into the whole health of baby and mother, which includes supporting and encouraging the breastfeeding relationship.

Community and Online Support

In the last chapter, I mentioned consulting with a local Infant Feeding Team when I was breastfeeding Philip. While my family was supportive and encouraging of breastfeeding my children, there were some obstacles we encountered that they weren't as familiar with navigating. I was fortunate enough to have the Infant Feeding Team to rely on for support and advice.

Thanks to our digital age and the increase in support for breastfeeding mothers, it has seemed to become easier than ever to discover different support groups for breastfeeding moms. If you're not sure where to start, different social media platforms like Facebook often have virtual groups you can join and ask questions if you have them. You can simply search for breastfeeding support in the city you live in. Some of these virtual groups may even have in-person meetups, which can be helpful if a hands-on approach would benefit you more.

Even if you don't experience any trials while breastfeeding, these support groups can be great to connect with other breastfeeding moms. It can be nice to share your experiences and feel validated if something seems weird to you, but you discover other moms have experienced it, too. Support groups can give new moms a sense of belonging and encouragement as they navigate new waters and get used to life with a new baby. Additionally, your experience may be what another mom needs to feel supported and encouraged. So, even if you have established a successful breastfeeding relationship, I would still encourage you to connect with a support group because you never know when you might need it or when someone might need you.

If you're not sure where to begin, I would recommend looking to the La Leche League. They're an international organization run by volunteers whose mission, according to their website, is "To help mothers worldwide to breastfeed through mother-to-mother support, encouragement, information, and education, and to promote a better understanding of breastfeeding as an important element in the healthy development of the baby and mother" (Philosophy, n.d.). They often have Facebook groups organized by geographical location, and these groups can inform you of in-person meetups. Usually (but, of course, it depends on the availability of the volunteers), they have monthly meetings where new mothers are encouraged to attend whether or not they're experiencing difficulty with breastfeeding. Their local groups often also have a leader whose phone number is shared publicly, so you can always call if you're experiencing an obstacle that you may need help with and that can't wait until an in-person meeting.

Whether it's online support groups or in-person meetings, I would highly recommend reaching out and finding a group for support to come alongside you as you acclimate to your new body and baby.

CONCLUSION

—◆—

I can only hope that my personal experiences can give you information about what to keep an eye out for and what to avoid as you embark on (or continue) your breastfeeding journey. It can be such a beautiful and natural relationship, but like many relationships, you're likely to hit some road bumps along the way.

Let this be a manual of sorts as you navigate these new roads of motherhood.

If you take anything away from this book, let it empower you to evaluate the relationship between you and your baby and make decisions that are best for the two of you and your family. Many people may try to weigh in and judge your decisions, but that's not their place. Don't hesitate to walk away from people who don't support and encourage your decisions when you're doing the best you can (sometimes, this can include medical professionals who aren't hearing you!).

Remember that whether this is your first baby or your fifth, each child is different, and each breastfeeding journey will be different as well. Embark on the journey with eyes wide open and an open mind that is receptive to understanding, empathetic, and nonjudgmental support from those around you. Whether that support comes from family, friends, or a support group you've sought out specifically for breastfeeding mothers, remember that it often takes a village to raise a child! We weren't meant to take this journey solo.

If you found this resource helpful, would you be so kind as to leave a review? Reviews help other readers know that this is a worthwhile book to have, and I would so appreciate you sharing your feedback!

About the Author

—◆—

Alicia lives in the leafy English countryside with her wonderful soon-to-be husband, four adored children, and three dogs. Country walks, adventures with the children, and curling up by the fire with a good book are all life essentials for Alicia.

Her days are filled with outdoor adventures, tending to her dogs and chickens, and savoring the joy of cooking delicious meals. Her sociable nature finds solace in coffee dates with friends, where she offers friendly, nonjudgmental advice and shares personal experiences, though she doesn't provide official medical guidance.

Through her book, Alicia aims to empower and support mothers on their individual breastfeeding journeys by providing a compassionate and empathetic perspective.

References

Breastfeeding - deciding when to stop. (2012). Better Health.
    https://www.betterhealth.vic.gov.au/health/Health
    yLiving/breastfeeding-deciding-when-to-stop

Cleveland Clinic. (2021, December 16). *Lactation (human milk
    production): Causes & how it works.*
    https://my.clevelandclinic.org/health/body/22201-
    lactation

Gurevich, R. (2019, November 12). *How to practice self-care as a
    new mom.* Verywell Family.
    https://www.verywellfamily.com/how-to-practice-
    self-care-as-a-new-mom-4771779

Infant food and feeding. (2021, July 6). American Academy of
    Pediatrics. https://www.aap.org/en/patient-
    care/healthy-active-living-for-families/infant-food-
    and-feeding/

Let-down reflex. (2022, May). Pregnancy Birth Baby.
    https://www.pregnancybirthbaby.org.au/let-down-
    reflex

Mullane, E. (2023, June 15). *Healthy breastfeeding diet, exercise
    and lifestyle.* Raising Children Network.
    https://raisingchildren.net.au/grown-ups/looking-
    after-yourself/new-mums/breastfeeding-diet-
    lifestyle

Philosophy. (n.d.). La Leche League International.
https://llli.org/about/philosophy/

Pope, A. (1727). *Letter to Gay.* Goodreads.
https://www.goodreads.com/quotes/36806-
blessed-is-he-who-expects-nothing-for-he-shall-
never

Wiessinger, D., West, D., Pitman, T., & La Leche League
International. (2010). *The womanly art of breastfeeding.*
Pinter & Martin.

World Health Organization. (2019). *Breastfeeding.*
https://www.who.int/health-
topics/breastfeeding#tab=tab_1